Commodities of Care

COMMODITIES OF CARE

The Business of HIV Testing in China

ELSA L. FAN

University of Minnesota Press
Minneapolis
London

Portions of chapters 2 and 3 are adapted from "HIV Testing as Prevention among MSM in China: The Business of Scaling-Up," *Global Public Health* 9, nos. 1–2 (2014): 85–97; reprinted by permission of the publisher, Taylor & Francis Ltd., http://www.tandfonline.com. Portions of chapters 2 and 3 and the Conclusion are adapted from "Counting Results: Performance-Based Financing and HIV Testing among MSM in China," *Critical Public Health* 27, no. 2 (2017): 217–27; reprinted by permission of the publisher, Taylor & Francis Ltd., http://www.tandfonline.com.

Published by the University of Minnesota Press
111 Third Avenue South, Suite 290
Minneapolis, MN 55401-2520
http://www.upress.umn.edu

ISBN 978-1-5179-0764-8 (hc)
ISBN 978-1-5179-0765-5 (pb)
Library of Congress record available at https://lccn.loc.gov/2021023191.

For my parents

CONTENTS

PREFACE

PARTS OF THIS BOOK were written during a turbulent and unprecedented moment in history, at least in my lifetime thus far: at the intersection of the COVID-19 pandemic, which has led to a reckoning of the role public health plays in our everyday lives, and the resurgence of the Black Lives Matter movement in the United States and globally. At such a time, it seems almost disingenuous to publish a book like this one, a book that appears critical of global public health. This book may be misinterpreted by some to undermine the widespread testing efforts that have become a cornerstone of the global public health response to the pandemic in which we currently find ourselves, at least at the time of this writing. And yet, I believe that to (mis)read this book in this way is to misunderstand my intentions.

First, it is important to point out, as some scholars have already done (see, e.g., Bulled and Singer 2020; Sangaramoorthy 2020), the parallels between the HIV epidemic in its nascent stages and COVID-19 today. At best, both have been characterized as "foreign" diseases that seek to penetrate and destroy populations (read white populations). We cannot forget still circulating understandings and associations of HIV as coming from the "dark continent" of Africa or the representations of this "savage" disease threatening to ravage white bodies. Such imagery matches the contemporary rhetoric, riddled with phrases like "kung flu" and the "Chinese virus," that too many speakers today use to describe COVID-19. To perpetuate these racially driven representations of the coronavirus is to blame certain populations for spreading the virus, and yet to accept their deaths.

At worst, the current pandemic has been fueled by conspiracy theories that it is a biological weapon deployed by China to weaken the Global North. Let us not forget similar conspiracy theories implicating HIV-positive people as intentionally spreading the virus to others by way of needles left in public spaces (the mall, movie theater seats, gas pumps, etc.). To be sure, the latter only underscores representations of HIV-positive people as certain kinds of people capable of doing certain kinds of things. COVID-19 similarly evoked early depictions of all

Asians as guilty. We cannot be naive enough to think that ideas of this nature are not intimately linked to and shaped by HIV as a disease of Africa or COVID-19 as a disease of China, thereby reproducing cultural narratives, as Paula Treichler (1999) noted, of disease and place being entwined or, as Susan Sontag (1989, 11) wrote, "envisaged as an alien 'other.'"

Second, it is worth asking, whose health matters? Already we have seen COVID-19 disproportionately affect black and brown bodies, just as HIV has impoverished the same communities both in the United States and globally. The cultural narratives underpinning HIV and COVID-19 intersect in crucial ways with the antiracist sentiments that fuel the Black Lives Matter movement. How and why do we continue to accept the unequal value humans place on differing bodies, an inequality that, though ever present, is made all the more visible, and palpable, in times of epidemics and pandemics? More importantly, how do we respond effectively to overcome and eradicate this injustice?

Let me be clear. In this book, I do not suggest, nor do I believe, that HIV testing or any testing should not be promoted or that it is ineffective; on the contrary, this technology is a critical part of a wider arsenal of strategies that is necessary to prevent and control epidemics and, for that matter, pandemics, as we are now all too aware. As I wrestled with how to reconcile my critiques at a time when science and public health were coming under attack, I had to remind myself that it is also science that tells us testing alone will not stem HIV, just as testing alone will not control COVID-19. Instead, I show, as many anthropologists before me have demonstrated, that testing and other interventions should be carried out within and as part of local health systems (see Biehl and Petryna 2013; Pfeiffer and Nichter 2008; Storeng 2014), but more importantly, they need to be understood as part of the social worlds that shape—and in which people make—important health decisions. As we have seen in the case of HIV, and as we will continue to see as things further unravel in the case of COVID-19, stemming an epidemic or a pandemic requires a multipronged response that must marshal the resources not only of public health and epidemiology but also of the social sciences, including anthropology.

To study the unexpected and often unanticipated effects of health interventions like testing men who have sex with men (MSM) in China and elsewhere is not to undermine scientific endeavors; by now, I hope it has been made abundantly clear how necessary knowledge born of scientific critique can be to the world. Rather, research like and including what I recount in the pages that follow demands that we acknowledge the fact that health in all of its forms—interventions, care, science, management, knowledge—does not operate independently of the systems and structures in which it is embedded or the social and cultural worlds in which we all live. These systems, and these worlds, affect how we carry out interventions, how we approach and treat disease, how we think about health, and whose health matters, writ large.

While the world, and the United States especially, struggles to contain the spread of COVID-19, we can only hope that we take history seriously and learn from it.

INTRODUCTION

"MEI NÜ!" (A TERM OF ENDEARMENT AMONG FRIENDS), called out Xiao Guo, as my colleague Zhang Li and I headed down the noisy street toward his office located in an urban metropolis of southern China.[1] I first met Xiao Guo in March 2011, during a workshop organized by the AIDS in China Fund (ACF), an American-based donor supporting HIV initiatives in China. The workshop was part of ACF's Test, Treat, and Prevent project, which had been designed to train staff and volunteers from community-based organizations to administer rapid HIV testing to men who have sex with men, or MSM. At the time, Xiao Guo was a college student attending the workshop on behalf of Guang Ai (hereinafter referred to as Bright Love), a local organization that provided sexual health services to youth and adolescent MSM and with which Xiao Guo volunteered part time.

A few months after our initial meeting, I traveled with Zhang Li, an officer with ACF, to visit Bright Love as one of our stops on a regional monitoring trip we were taking to check in with ACF's grantees, and it was Xiao Guo, exuding enthusiasm, who greeted us when we arrived on that blustery autumn day. He gave us a tour of Bright Love's new office space, then located inside a multistory white building tucked away in a small pocket of buildings off a main road and underneath a sprawling labyrinth of highways. I could hear the cars whizzing by above us, a reminder of how quickly things moved in China. Once we were inside the building, Xiao Guo proudly showed off the pristine rooms where he and others at Bright Love planned and hosted events for college students—the organization's target demographic. In addition to their in-house events held at the office, Bright Love implemented outreach activities in and around local universities, and it was these activities that motivated the organization's recent move: the new site was just a few miles away from a local university.

"This is the activity room," said Xiao Guo as we entered into an open space where they hosted dance parties, movie nights, and more. These types of events, he explained, performed triple duty by serving as a way to educate participants about sexual health and HIV/STI (sexually transmitted infection) prevention, advertise the organization's testing services, and provide a safe social space for MSM to get together and interact. Bright Love's involvement with ACF's Test, Treat, and Prevent project to scale up HIV testing among MSM, which I describe in later chapters, provided the material support to carry out the organization's testing services.

As we made our way in and out of and up and down the different rooms inside the multistory building, we came upon a "lounge area," as Xiao Guo called it, a spacious room populated with colorful sofas and chairs and a coffee table covered with various magazines and other reading materials. Laid visibly atop the table were several multicolored, laminated sheets of paper. Xiao Guo picked up one of the sheets and handed it to Zhang Li and me, explaining as he did so, "We put this together to give to clients [*kehu*, the word he used to refer to men who came in for HIV testing]." The laminated paper detailed the pricing for Bright Love's HIV testing services. "We typically do rapid HIV testing [*kuaijian*] by appointment only, and we limit those services to Fridays, Saturdays, and Sundays," he described; "for each HIV test, we charge 20 Chinese yuan [CNY; USD 3], but we call it an 'operating cost' [*chengben feiyong*], rather than a 'fee.'"[2]

In addition to ACF's testing project, Xiao Guo informed us, Bright Love participated in other HIV initiatives oriented around testing MSM, including those managed by the Health Fund and the Global Fund to Fight AIDS, Tuberculosis and Malaria (the Global Fund), two more global health donors operating in China. Unlike ACF's project, which provided material rather than financial support to community-based organizations, the Health Fund and the Global Fund adopted performance-based financing schemes that tied payments in the form of performance incentives to the delivery of performance targets. Xiao Guo admitted that for the Health Fund in particular, Bright Love primarily recruited and referred MSM to the local Chinese Center for Disease Control (CDC)—the nation's public health arm—to get tested for HIV. In return, Bright Love received incentives for each person tested for HIV, each HIV-positive case detected, and other predetermined outputs. He noted that if a person tests positive from the rapid HIV tests provided by ACF (as part of the Test, Treat, and Prevent project), Bright Love then refers this person to the CDC to get retested and thereby collects additional incentives from the Health Fund. As

Xiao Guo described this process, he joked to us, "We are basically just selling blood [*mai xue*]."

Zhang Li asked about the status of ACF's project, since that was the reason for our visit, and whether Bright Love had identified any new cases since starting the project. We expected the answer to be yes, as had been the case with most of ACF's grantees participating in the project, but we did not expect the story we were about to hear. Xiao Guo responded that "actually, just the other day, three out of the four men who came into our office to get tested turned out to be HIV-positive." I must have looked as surprised as Zhang Li, who immediately exclaimed, "What? How did that happen?" Xiao Guo hesitated for a moment, looked away, slightly embarrassed, and then replied somewhat defensively, "OK, I'll tell you, but don't you heterosexuals [*yixinglian*] judge me." He continued:

> I was in an online tongzhi chat room and learned about an orgy that someone was organizing that weekend. Sometimes a person, usually someone rich, will rent out a hotel room or similar space for these things. I decided to go with a few of my friends; while there, we went around handing out condoms to people and telling them about our HIV testing services. We made a couple of new "friends" [*pengyou*] and encouraged them to come to our organization to get tested.[3] The next day, four of them came in to get tested, and three of them turned out to be HIV-positive.

＊ ＊ ＊ ＊ ＊

This book tells the story of how one health intervention—HIV testing among MSM—unfolded in the lives and communities of same-sex-desiring men in China. At the time of my fieldwork, the push to scale up this intervention became the dominant strategy par excellence to reduce HIV transmission in the hope of controlling the epidemic in the country; the intervention arrived at a moment of emerging crisis in the HIV epidemic that came to shape, in intimate ways, the lives of Chinese MSM. This book examines how the lives, and, in many cases, the livelihoods, of these men became sutured to HIV. This linkage reconfigured who the men were, how they understood themselves to be, and the possibilities for and limitations on who they could become. At the same time, this book provides a snapshot of the wider trends in global health programs that have shaped HIV interventions in China as elsewhere, radically altering the ways that health, disease, and even patients were, and continue to be, envisioned—as commodities, as data, and as things more generally.

These trends are nothing new. Medical anthropologists have long demonstrated how the very concept of health is intertwined with the accumulation of wealth, such as growing pharmaceutical markets across global spaces by way of drug development, biotechnologies, or clinical trials that capitalize on individual and mass health (Cooper and Waldby 2014; Dumit 2012; Petryna 2009; see also Sunder Rajan 2006), or, as other scholars have examined, how the circulation and commercialization of "tissue economies" (Waldby and Mitchell 2006) have generated new forms of life alongside new forms of prosperity (see also Song 2017). And yet, as I describe in this book, these trends animate new things. In the chapters that follow, I examine how HIV testing intersects with the lives of the people and communities targeted by this intervention. I argue that HIV testing targeted at and marketed to MSM transformed these men from subjects of care, whereby they were cared for as patients, into commodities of care, whereby they were transacted as economic and political capital. This transformation was made possible, I suggest, by "making up" (Hacking 1986) MSM as a new form of selfhood and subjectivity that men came to inhabit. By linking trends in global health to the production of MSM selfhoods and socialities that did not previously exist, this book makes clear the ways in which one particular health intervention—the scaling up of MSM testing—traveled, and also unraveled, across social and cultural contexts in unexpected ways.

*   *   *   *   *

I began with Xiao Guo's story because it is one that became familiar to me over the course of my research. A significant portion of my fieldwork involved traveling around the country to meet with staff and volunteers of MSM organizations involved with HIV testing initiatives and with men who were tested as a part of these projects. When I arrived in 2010 for my extended fieldwork, the link between MSM and HIV had already been solidified, such that any organization serving these men included a component of, if not entirely dedicating their services to, testing this population. That is to say, HIV and MSM were inextricably intertwined. In my travels, I met with dozens of organizations that were consistently discovering new HIV-positive MSM, much as Xiao Guo and Bright Love did. The detection of HIV among these men became so alarmingly frequent that my colleagues' and my questions for community-based organizations shifted quickly from whether they had identified new HIV cases to *how many cases* they had identified.

As I traveled the country, I became acutely aware of the complex and contradictory scenarios evoked by scaling up MSM testing. I listened to the experiences of men who had just discovered they were HIV-positive, as they struggled to reconcile their newfound statuses with their same-sex desires and societal pressures for heteronormativity. I attended meetings with public health officials who debated how to address rising HIV rates among MSM to curtail the epidemic, while simultaneously implementing interventions that had the potential to undercut those aims. I worked with donors who prioritized short-term, cost-effective strategies, often at the expense of longer-term, more comprehensive approaches to reducing HIV transmission. Several times, I was unwittingly drawn into political battles among community-based organizations as they struggled to stay afloat financially, even as they criticized others for utilizing similar tactics to survive. I observed bitter rivalries play out around the use of performance-based financing and other forms of incentivization—such as charging for HIV testing, as Bright Love did—as a consequence of dwindling HIV resources. These rivalries pitted people, and entire communities, against one another, undermining wider advocacy efforts for MSM. Although at times, the drive to reduce HIV among MSM seemed to be the anchor for bringing disparate players together, in other moments, it was the very thing wedging them apart.

This book traces the movement of HIV testing across all these scenarios and analyzes its impacts as a health technology as it intersects with two key themes I describe in these chapters. First is how audit cultures (Strathern 2000) governing health programs are (re)shaping the way prevention and control are administered. The privileging of technical interventions like testing and vertical initiatives by global health donors allows for the kind of accounting and accountability measures that most donors now favor. Language such as "value for money," "return on investment," and "cost-effectiveness" are no longer just descriptors of health interventions; these concepts are increasingly becoming the architects of them. The yoking of MSM testing to accountability mechanisms like performance-based financing promised, on one hand, to align health and financial outcomes and, on the other, to ensure donors a more transparent accounting of how their money is being spent. This intervention reveals how deeply audit regimes have taken hold and reconfigured the landscape of HIV prevention and care—a landscape that, as I describe in this book, relies not only on locating but on making up MSM.

This making up of MSM leads to the second theme I explore in this book: how audit regimes are shifting the way the MSM category is "transformed, reinvented, reworked, and reimagined" (Parker 2019, 271), which in turn inspires new ways for donors, public health professionals, and community-based organizations to think about, mobilize, and measure this population. I show how this MSM testing intervention has led to new social formations, new identity politics, and new ways for men who desire and have sex with other men to understand themselves as MSM. I suggest that the socially constructed, shared understanding that MSM are almost always already infected with HIV as a result of their same-sex sexual practices stoked public health anxieties around the "hiddenness" of the population in China, as many MSM are married to women. These discourses presented MSM as a category and as a community that must be intervened upon as scientific object. These same discourses propelled MSM to take action for themselves as sexual subjects. As I illustrate throughout this book, people do not just inhabit categories; categories presuppose people.

By tracing the circulation of HIV testing across bodies and spaces, I attend to what this testing technology does, and what it enables, as it travels: eliciting HIV statuses, standardizing MSM, evoking new selfhoods and socialities, generating profits, and reshaping understandings of proper conduct. Around this technology are possibilities for people to count and to be counted. Indeed, if there is one story that unexpectedly emerges in this book, and yet recedes into the shadows, it is that of the productivity of the HIV test.

GLOBAL HEALTH FINANCING, AUDIT CULTURES, AND THE PROMISE OF HIV TESTING

How did HIV testing, and the scale-up of testing, become such a prominent part of the public health landscape in China? How did this intervention travel across communities of MSM, and what did it leave in its wake? These are just some of the questions that drive this book, as I describe in the following chapters. To truly appreciate the impacts, and implications, of this intervention as it unfolded across the country, let us first turn to the wider context in which HIV testing among MSM gained traction not just in China but as part of a wider shift in global health. This requires attending to the financial flows that increasingly govern health programs.

As I noted in my opening paragraph, I met Xiao Guo at one of ACF's quarterly workshops organized for its grantees involved with the Test, Treat, and Prevent project. During the three-day event, we covered a range of topics related to MSM testing, including the prospect of charging "clients" for HIV testing services offered by community-based organizations, a practice that Bright Love adopted. It quickly became clear to me over the course of the workshop that Bright Love, along with many other grantees, was involved not only with ACF's project but also with multiple other testing initiatives operating in the country, all targeting MSM for testing. One of these initiatives was an HIV program administered by the Health Fund, the other donor whose MSM testing endeavors I discuss in this book.[4]

As I followed the testing initiatives of these two donors (ACF and the Health Fund) during my fieldwork, I started to realize just how powerful this intervention had become in shaping and interacting with existing local public health responses to the epidemic, particularly in regard to MSM. For Bright Love and other community-based organizations involved with providing HIV services, the predominance of testing and the incentives attached to it became an economic lifeline, especially as the international HIV donors that these organizations relied so heavily upon began to withdraw from the country. Bright Love's activities organized around mobilizing MSM to get tested made a new kind of sense, because doing so allowed the organization to survive financially. Bright Love represents the many organizations I came to know and describe in this book whose work gradually coalesced around recruiting men to get tested just as the kinds of prevention and care available to MSM slowly narrowed. The prevalence of testing MSM as a key prevention strategy signaled a new trajectory for controlling the epidemic in China, one that favored a magic-bullet approach that divorced technical interventions from the wider social worlds in which they were administered.

The entrenchment of this testing intervention in China cannot be understood outside of the international networks and financial flows that direct it. Prior to 2003, most national HIV and AIDS programs in the country were supported and shaped by international donors. From 1988 to 2009, international support accounted for nearly one-third of the total funding for all HIV programs in the country (Sun et al. 2010). Needless to say, these donors made a tremendous impact in galvanizing the government to take action to address the epidemic not only by providing financial resources but also by introducing international best practices. For instance, efforts by bilateral and multilateral institutions like the World Health Organization (WHO) and the World Bank were instrumental in setting up and strengthening HIV surveillance systems. Donors helped to improve the government's capacity to implement and innovate national AIDS programs (Wu et al. 2011). In earlier stages of the epidemic, international funders introduced key interventions and strategies to prevent HIV in specific population groups, such as condom promotion and on-site STI clinics for sex workers and methadone-maintenance clinics for people who inject drugs. Perhaps no other institution had a greater impact on addressing the epidemic in China than the Global Fund, which has contributed more than USD 300 million alone to HIV and AIDS since 2004 (Global Fund 2020).[5]

Donors also drew attention to MSM as a key population to address. Until the mid-2000s, MSM remained largely marginal to the national HIV response, and the group was only added to national sentinel surveillance activities in 2003 (Jia et al. 2007) despite the growing visibility of gay and lesbian culture throughout the 1990s, especially in China's urban centers (Ho 2010; Rofel 1999). Any attention to MSM came primarily at the behest of international donors. For instance, the first government-initiated intervention for MSM came by way of support from the United Kingdom's Department for International Development in 2002, and a subsequent sixty-one-city survey of MSM in 2008–9 was carried out with the support of the Bill and Melinda Gates Foundation (the Gates Foundation) (Sun et al. 2010). Bright Love, along with other community-based organizations, greatly benefited from this newfound attention to MSM.

The abundance of HIV resources in China at that time tracks loosely with a wider uptick in development assistance for health globally in roughly the same period, growing at an average rate of 10.03 percent annually between 2000 and 2010 (Chang et al. 2019). This surge has been attributed to a new cohort of global health players, including the Global Fund, the Vaccine Alliance (Gavi), and, most notably, the Gates Foundation. These players are credited with ushering in alternative ways of thinking about and acting upon disease, prioritizing the use of business logics and practices to address health needs. These shifts have translated into a narrower mandate that privileges technical interventions and vertical disease-specific initiatives that are mobile, portable, and scalable, thereby catering readily to the delivery of economic metrics and allowing donors to better account for health spending. The Gates Foundation in particular has made unprecedented strides in transforming the global health landscape, shaping regional, national, and international agendas by way of decisions about where, how, and what to support with its vast resources (McCoy, Chand, and Sridhar 2009; Sridhar and Craig 2011). A recent study in the *Lancet* shows how these financing flows are leading global health governance toward the interests of a handful of donors whose extensive discretionary funding plus business logics have privileged short-term, vertical programs at the expense of longer-term health system strengthening (Clinton and Sridhar 2017b; see also Storeng 2014).

The scope and scale of these trends have certainly been felt as donors have made their way into China. The practices favored by global health donors gradually came to intersect with the culture of HIV and public health programs in China. I recall hearing, for instance, a program officer for the Health Fund explain the need for performance metrics to community-based organizations: "Impact should be measured by *actual* performance, not just by saying you did the job." Not only did her statement communicate the distrust of these organizations by donors (as I detail in chapter 1); it also underlined the rationale behind the use of accountability measures like performance-based financing, that is, to hold organizations answerable for how they spent donor money. As I illustrate, MSM testing and its attachment to performance-based financing allowed donors and other stakeholders closer monitoring of their funding, giving them the flexibility to quickly redirect their resources toward recipients that deliver cost-effectiveness and meet performance goals, and away from those who do not, even at the expense of actual health. This approach consolidated the public health need to deliver evidence-based interventions. As Susan Erikson (2016, 148) argued, accountability metrics are more and more sutured to "market metrics and logics" on the assumption that better financial outcomes lead to better health outcomes. This is a premise I question throughout the book. Health, Erikson suggests, becomes redefined not as a thing to be improved per se but as an investment that must generate a return. As a consequence, organizations like Bright Love increasingly adapted their activities toward meeting donor, rather than community, needs.

The demand for financial accountability explains, then, the penchant for technical solutions (e.g., drugs, vaccines, HIV testing) by these "newer" global health actors. On one hand, such approaches offer the kinds of results that deliver economic and scientific returns. As a consultant working with a global health donor in China once explained to me when I asked why they invested in MSM rather than general prevention work, "this is a results-based program, so we need to see indicators and deliverables. Besides, how would you measure success in the general population?"

But on the other hand, technical solutions tend to be divorced from their social and cultural contexts and take as a given local experiences and behaviors (Birn 2005). As Adriana Petryna (2009) argued of standardized ethical guidelines in global clinical trials, they often fail to take into consideration constraints and other factors that might influence a participant's decision to take part in such trials. Far from being voluntary, participants often see trials as the only or best way to meet their health needs, even if temporarily, because many are unlikely to be able to afford expensive treatments outside of the trials. Petryna draws our attention to how participation itself cannot be separated from why people enroll in the first place. In much the same way, the discourse and practice of HIV testing among MSM disassociate the act of getting tested from how men came to be infected with HIV. I suggest that linking performance-based financing and other forms of incentivization to testing has almost ensured, in the case of MSM in China at the time of my fieldwork, that only men were getting tested, and that men were only getting tested. While this was not true of all HIV testing initiatives, an unexpected effect of the HIV intervention promoted by donors was a very narrow purview of what mattered, and this left little room, or funding, to explore alternative methods of prevention and care for MSM.

It is worth remembering that the inclusion of business rationales in global health programs is not new. As Linsey McGoey (2016) explained, these ideas and practices were present long before the buzzwords we now use for them appeared in the field. But what *is* new, she argued, is the scale and speed at which business approaches are being deployed, along with the explicitness of self-interest and for-profit ends toward which health programs are being implemented. Bright Love, after all, made no secret of its participation in multiple testing initiatives, nor did it see any conflict with charging fees for its testing services while using ACF's materials to claim incentives from the Health Fund's program. Rather than seeing these acts as incongruous, I argue that their practices are perfectly aligned with the business logics and rationales that guide interventions like scaling up MSM testing. These interventions enable, and perhaps even require, that stakeholders (donors, service providers) see the generation of profit as vital to effective and efficient health service provision. That is to say, profit now seems to be an entitlement. An HIV activist once asked in a meeting during a debate around organizations charging for HIV testing, "If people are willing to pay for it, why shouldn't you charge for your services?" This and similar attitudes are especially acute when they come to bear on setting global health agendas and priorities that might affect the most in need of health gains, yet promise the lowest financial gains.

IMAGINING, AND TESTING MSM

The turn to scaling up MSM testing, I argue in this book, animated new ways for MSM to imagine themselves and their same-sex desires, but also new ways for these men to be imagined by donors and other stakeholders (e.g., public health authorities). At the same time, the catalyst for testing MSM came partly out of imaginations of these men as certain kinds of people. Therefore how MSM were seen, or not, in global and national HIV strategies had everything to do with *how* they were seen as a key population (Biruk 2012; McKay 2016; see also Scott 1998).

The MSM category originated out of a public health need for epidemiological surveillance, not as an identity category around which men identify and therefore can be mobilized into action (such as "gay"). However, this category's focus on sexual behavior quickly came under fire for its narrow purview of HIV risk.[6] Rebecca Young and Ilan Meyer (2005), for instance, pointed out that MSM as a category is predicated on mainly Euro-American assumptions of concordance between sexuality, desire, and behavior; as such, it obscures important dimensions of sexuality that may impact HIV transmission. Their critique was supported by findings from other scholars who underscored the limitations to adopting a strictly behavior-based category, including marginalizing sexual minorities that may be equally vulnerable to HIV and ignoring the needs of diverse subgroups within HIV programs (Carrillo and Hoffman 2016; Muñoz-Laboy 2004; see also Parker, Aggleton, and Perez-Brumer 2016).

Beyond these programmatic critiques, however, lay a more pernicious outcome of the MSM category: the separation of "gay" from "MSM." The original intent behind creating "MSM" was to distinguish MSM from gay to lessen the stigmatizing effects around identity, especially because scientists had classified "gay" as an HIV risk (an early acronym for HIV was GRID, for "gay-related immune deficiency"). The possibility that there were men who did not identify as gay or passed as heterosexual but who also had sex with men prompted public health concerns that HIV could become a generalized epidemic, one not limited to specific subpopulations. The MSM category, as an epidemiological instrument, attempted to counteract these effects by focusing on behavior only, in the hope of rendering these men more thinkable, as well as intervenable, casting them as behavioral objects isolated from social worlds rather than as sexual subjects embedded in these social worlds, for the purposes of HIV surveillance (see Boellstorff 2011). Instead, the separation of gay (as identity) and MSM (as behavior) only reproduced representations of the latter as dangerous and illicit that took on racialized undertones (Gosine 2009).

Anthropologists have long examined how sexuality is made into an object of analysis through medicalization and pathologization (Adams and Pigg 2005). In China, this process developed out of an incursion of Western sexology. Historically, sexuality was considered an integral part of holistic life rather than a separate domain of activity, and it was deeply tied to one's kinship system (Chou 2000, 2001). As a result, same-sex relations were tolerated so long as they did not disrupt the social and political order and a man fulfilled his filial and family responsibilities as a husband and father (Jeffreys and Yu 2015; Zheng 2015), an expectation that remains to this day. In the 1920s, terms such as *tongxinglian'ai* and *tongxing'ai,* translated directly from English texts, came into use to describe homosexual relations (Kang 2010). These terms pathologized homosexuality as a sexual perversion, thereby transforming same-sex sexual behaviors into an object of scientific inquiry. The inclusion of homosexuality as a sexual disorder into the Chinese Classification of Mental Disorders further entrenched sexuality as a "thing one administered" (Foucault 1978, 24; see also Dikötter 1995).[7] As Travis Kong (2016, 500) wrote, "from the 1900s to 1979, a dominant sexological construction of the homosexual subject was constructed as the 'other'—as a sexual perversion to be cured, as a violation of the heterosexual order to be silenced, or as a threat to patriarchal order to be regulated." In short, same-sex relations transitioned from a tolerated social practice into a medicalized sexual perversion that needed to be policed, along with the men who engaged in these acts.

The regulation of sexuality, in China and elsewhere, took a significant turn as a result of the global HIV epidemic. Sexuality was propelled to the forefront of the epidemic response, and the need to regulate it was recast as a matter of disease transmission control. That is to say, questions about who had sex with whom as a personal matter gave way to more medical and scientific framings regarding how the virus spread through sexual activity (Pigg and Adams 2005, 19). In turn, certain people and their sexual practices were transformed into "risk groups" or "key populations" to be sorted, counted, surveilled, and deemed dangerous for, or in danger of, transmitting and contracting the virus. MSM reflected these risks eminently, not as men having sex with other men, but rather as men more likely to spread HIV to other men via anal sex and to women because of their "denial of," as is often said, their "true" sexual identity.

Indeed, interventions that target people's sex lives are shaped by presumptions of what people do sexually and how they should behave morally, something to which Xiao Guo was no doubt attuned when he asked us "heterosexuals" (Zhang Li and I) not to judge him before recounting his story about intervening in an orgy for MSM. They work to reinforce what we think we already know about people and places. As I show in this book, Euro-American notions of sexuality that inform most international interventions are especially ill suited to the Chinese context. An estimated one-third (Gao, Zhang, and Jin 2009) to one-half (Han et al. 2016) of MSM in China are likely to be married due to the strong social and cultural values accorded to heterosexual marriage. Chinese MSM's sexual "transgressions" of non-Chinese models of sexuality tend to render them as sexual deviants who require regulatory interventions, if not by the state, then by international agencies (Gosine 2009). In this way, the imagination of who MSM are and what they do converges with questions about what to do with these men because of who they are or are imagined to be.

By the time I arrived in China in 2010, a key development in the HIV sector made it possible for testing to take hold: sexual contact overtook intravenous drug use as the leading route of HIV transmission in the mid-2000s. The epidemiological shift invited increased scrutiny of MSM, which was guided by the assumption that many of the men counted in the data identified as heterosexual but engaged in same-sex sexual practices. It is more than likely that the men targeted by Xiao Guo and his colleagues at the male orgy were of this demographic, because attending hidden events minimizes the risk that men's same-sex sexual activities will be exposed.

The expansion of HIV testing among Chinese MSM can be read as a response to the problem of identifying married men who have sex with other men. This intervention, I argue in this book, anticipates and "demands *kinds* of things or people to count" (Hacking 1982, 280) that may not have been countable before. Thus testing arose partly out of a general need to test, detect, and surveil MSM, especially HIV-positive men, to reduce transmission (see chapter 2). And yet, MSM required a different sort of intervention than those targeting identifiable populations like sex workers and people who inject drugs; that is, they needed an approach in which men could be mobilized to seek out testing services on their own despite their double lives and complex social and sexual lifestyles.

THE TRANSFORMATION AND COMMODIFICATION OF MSM

How does one come to get tested as an MSM? How is it that the men tested by Bright Love came to be tested at all? Did they learn to conceive of themselves as at risk for HIV before choosing to get tested? If so, how did they learn? The activities carried out by Bright Love, from hosting movie nights to intervening in male orgies, were typical of the kinds of outreach that community-based organizations conducted to mobilize MSM to get tested as part of wider MSM testing initiatives.

Bright Love never specifically targeted MSM per se in its activities, nor did the men it targeted in its activities explicitly identify as "MSM." Nevertheless, these men came to be included under and counted as MSM in testing initiatives regardless of their sexual identities, preferences, and lifestyles.

By and into the 2000s, understandings of MSM as a category evolved, shifting away from its original focus on sexual behavior only and expanding to include gay men and other sexual orientations. For example, a UNAIDS (2006) report defined MSM as "any man who has sex with a man, thus accommodating a variety of sexual identities as well as those who do not self-identify as homosexual or gay." Soon after, the Foundation for AIDS Research (amfAR; 2008, 5) added "male sex workers, transgendered people, and a range of culture- and country-specific populations of MSM" to the category. The men I came to know in China, and whom I describe in this book, represented a wide array of sexual orientations including *tongzhi* (emic term to index same-sex desire), *gay* (in English), *tongxinglian* (medicalized term for homosexual), and others. As sociologist Sun Zhongxin and others (2006, 11) stated in their study of Chinese MSM, "our findings indicate that there is no single accepted term for identifying a male homosexual sexual orientation among MSM in Shanghai. Men use a variety of terms, primarily *tongzhi*, 'gay,' *quanneiren* and *tongxinglian*." Similarly, a report published by USAID and Family Health International (n.d., 42) used *MSM* and *tongzhi* interchangeably, noting that the men in their study "used a range of terms to describe their same sex behaviors and identities."

In this book, I use *MSM* rather than *tongzhi, gay* (in English), or any of the preceding terms because *MSM* is the language used by my interlocutors to describe the men they serve and because the men they serve did not always adopt same-sex sexual identities. But also, I employ *MSM* because I am interested in how understandings of this category have changed in relation to the testing interventions I examine in this book and that I argue compelled Xiao Guo and others like him to "make up" MSM to mobilize more men to get tested for HIV on their own, much like the men who came into his office the day after the orgy to get tested. Ian Hacking (1986) demonstrated how making up people is intimately linked to statistical science and the need to count and classify people. As I show in the following chapters, making up MSM emerged out of a need to count these men in the testing initiatives, like those of ACF and the Health Fund, described in this book. By making up MSM, I index two things. First, I refer to the process of cultivating in men who engage in sexual activities with other men a selfhood by which they came to recognize their same-sex desires and their HIV risk as part and parcel to their same-sex sexual practices as MSM. I am therefore interested less in men adopting an MSM identity than I am in how same-sex-desiring men, regardless of their sexual identity or lifestyles, come to inhabit an MSM subject position as HIV risky. A key question I ask in this book, then, is, in what ways has HIV testing reshaped how these men come to understand themselves, and to understand themselves as almost always already infected with HIV? I show how the targeting of these men for HIV testing has enabled new and increasingly complex forms of selfhood and community to transpire. These shifts, in turn, instantiate a subject position from which men learn to accept their same-sex desires as sutured to HIV risk.

Second, I refer to the practices of enumeration that facilitate the emergence of an MSM selfhood. The push to scale up MSM testing hinges on the existence of a population *to* test or, at the very least, on the possibility of creating a community of men able to be mobilized to get tested. The testing initiatives I describe, such as the ones in which Bright Love participated, provided monetary incentives for testing MSM and additional rewards for detecting new HIV cases. These performance incentives, I argue, reorganized the value of MSM bodies and transformed them into commodities of care. In the context of performance metrics, what came to matter was not just if or how men identified as MSM but also how they were counted as MSM to meet the performance targets attached to incentives.

Commodification, states Lesley Sharp (2000, 293), "insists upon objectification in some form, transforming persons and their bodies from a human category into objects of economic desire." Bodies must be dehumanized, severed in some way from any sense of personhood, whether they are medicalized into biological entities or fragmented into individual parts (e.g., their organs). The scale-up of MSM testing in China, especially as it became entangled with performance-based financing, made this process possible insofar as these bodies became treated as valuable, but scarce, resources that were economically coveted and could be exchanged for monetary incentives or for political capital that ensured some measure of financial stability for organizations (see chapter 3). Surely this outcome was not the intention behind MSM testing, and yet I show how testing unintentionally configured MSM as objects to be tested and transacted as economic and political capital rather than as men in need of care and support.

The incentives further accorded hierarchical values to different types of MSM bodies. As Xiao Guo explained, Bright Love received an additional incentive for every person who was confirmed to be HIV-positive and another incentive for each person who underwent a routine CD4 test used to determine the need for antiretroviral therapy (ART). In many cases, the amount provided for the detection of an HIV case was significantly higher than that given for testing alone. This differential pricing echoes the long history of commodifying bodies in the medical sphere that has often rendered dead bodies of greater value than living ones or, in this case, "diseased" bodies of greater value than healthy ones. It is not unusual for socially expendable bodies to accrue value through their participation in medical projects, such as global clinical trials (see Petryna 2009; Sunder Rajan 2007). MSM, a historically marginalized population that has acquired new forms of value through global and national HIV strategies that target their bodies are just another example. In this regard, the rendering of MSM bodies into commodities of care could almost be read as a logical outcome of the technical interventions—like scaling up MSM testing—that have been favored and prioritized by global health donors.

In this book, I demonstrate how MSM, as a category and as a community, has taken on new and varied meanings in direct response to health interventions, such as HIV testing among Chinese MSM. Already, scholars are starting to explore how the category "MSM" animates new things, people, spaces, and communities (see Boellstorff 2011; Fan, Thomann, and Lorway 2019). I show that MSM needed to be made legible to policy makers and donors, and HIV testing accomplished that goal by inscribing all MSM as risky.

SERENDIPITY AND ETHNOGRAPHIC ENCOUNTERS

This ethnography is the outcome of a series of unanticipated, and serendipitous, encounters.[8] The research on which it is based was carried out over a period of twenty-one months between 2008 and 2015. I conducted the bulk of my fieldwork in 2010 to 2011, while based out of Beijing, China, with shorter, supplementary visits during the summers in other years. I did not embark on a project to study HIV testing in MSM when I arrived in 2010. Rather, I had planned to study the makings of biosocial citizenship among former blood and plasma donors in rural, central China (see Asia Catalyst 2007; Rosenthal 2000, 2001). It was through moments of serendipity that I found myself "follow[ing] the thing" (Marcus 1995)—HIV testing—which led me to this project.

A pivotal moment was when I was invited by an acquaintance, who subsequently turned out to be one of my primary interlocutors, to a workshop he was facilitating for MSM in Beijing. I attended the event because I had nothing planned for that evening, unaware that this experience would come to alter the trajectory of my research. I spent the evening immersed in intimate discussions with men regarding their sexual experiences, working through how those experiences shaped their understandings of HIV risk in deeply personal, and unexpected, ways. Perhaps my most memorable takeaway from this night was how HIV permeated so many aspects of the lives of these men, from their sexual subjectivity to their sexual ethics.

As I began to follow the thread of HIV testing among MSM, I grew interested in how seemingly disparate things, in fact, were deeply entangled and contingent: how community-based organizations came to the forefront of this HIV intervention; how one health intervention shaped the contours of HIV prevention in public health; how exclusions became mapped along axes of morality and money; and how monetary incentives became crucial to carrying out HIV prevention work. Over time, I came to understand how a deceptively simple HIV intervention evolved to mean so much more to the men with whom I worked, animating radical shifts in individual subjectivities as well as the culture of health and disease in China.

Finally, it was serendipitous for me that this book came to fruition at all, because I almost missed the opportunity to attend graduate school. At the time of my acceptance, I had just moved back to the United States after spending years living in Asia and working in the development sector there, and I was merely days into a new position at a philanthropic organization. Were it not for my decision, paired with the generous support of my program in allowing me to defer my studies for a year to remain at that job, I might never have become interested in the kinds of ideological shifts already under way in the philanthropy world in which I was embedded. Those shifts mirrored, to a large extent, the market- and profit-oriented trends in global health that I explore in this book. Indeed, it was my time spent outside of academia that ultimately shaped my interests within it.

* * * * *

To follow HIV testing as a methodological strategy, I volunteered with three different institutions for my fieldwork. They provided me multiple, if not contradictory, perspectives on the design, implementation, and effects of this intervention. My decision to work with diverse groups, rather than embedding myself in just one, was motivated by my desire to trace the social, political, and biographical lives of HIV testing. As Arjun Appadurai (1986, 5) reminded us, "we have to follow the things themselves, for their meanings are inscribed in their forms, their uses, their trajectories." Locating myself at manifold sites allowed me to witness how a multiplicity of variously positioned people interacted with and gave meaning to this technology.

I spent the most time with ACF, a U.S.-based foundation supporting MSM-focused HIV prevention projects through small-scale grants and initiatives in China. ACF is not a large organization and has been supported over the years by a small group of loyal donors in the United States. It is an organization that is, in every sense of the word, grassroots. Despite limited resources, it has made important contributions to HIV work in no small part because of the networks cultivated by its director, Jonah, who split his time between the United States and China. As I discovered, Jonah both seemed to know everyone to know and was in the know about everything in the HIV sector in China, qualities that worked to my advantage. Because of ACF's work at the grassroots level, I was able to spend time with grassroots groups and the men they served, to gain a deeper perspective of the impacts HIV testing had on the lives of MSM and their communities.

My participation with ACF generally consisted of attending its activities, through which I came to know a handful of community-based organizations involved with MSM testing. Although I did not take part in designing or implementing their initiatives, I was part of many conversations with Jonah and Zhang Li, part of ACF's program team, to discuss issues that arose within their projects. I traveled extensively with ACF on many occasions as its representatives visited grantees.

These excursions provided perhaps the most insightful moments of my fieldwork. Ethnography, Stacy Leigh Pigg (2013, 132) wrote, is paying attention to "what falls out of view or falls between the cracks," and certainly, those moments of routine—waiting for the train, riding in taxis or on subway cars, and drawn-out meals in between—became unexpectedly vital.

I also volunteered with the Health Fund, an international organization supporting HIV prevention programs that included HIV testing among MSM in China, and their government counterpart administering the Health Fund's programs because international funding must be filtered through national and local government channels in China (Hildebrandt 2011). My work with these institutions provided me different perspectives into the decision-making rationales of donors and the kinds of tensions that shape policies and policy making. Far from consensual, the design and implementation of HIV programs were often the result of extended, and at times acrimonious, discussions negotiated under the guise of participation (Mosse 2003). Certainly the stakeholders in these programs did not always share end goals, and my time spent with them served as a reminder that institutions are fractious because they are made up of people with their own ideas, beliefs, and priorities that are never detached from the work they do. In this respect, I conducted a kind of "insider ethnography" (Vernooij 2017) that reveals the social actors behind the social institutions.

At times, my involvement was limited to observation, but I also transgressed the role of observer by participating in program activities. As George Marcus (1995) noted, ethnographers can be multipositioned as well as multisited. I quickly learned that my years of working as a development professional gave me more traction in the field than my association with an American university. And my interlocutors frequently leveraged that background for their own purposes. Therefore, as many anthropologists before me have found (Farmer 1992; Nguyen 2010), my presence often blurred the boundaries between researcher–participant–observer–practitioner. This meant that in addition to traveling with organizations on monitoring trips, I helped to evaluate and make recommendations on project proposals and funding requests, assisted in organizing workshops on HIV-related topics, and attended meetings at which programmatic decisions were made.

Indeed, I vacillated between the work of critically analyzing the things I did and participating in the very practices that I was meant to be, at least in theory, critically analyzing.

OVERVIEW OF THE BOOK

This book emerges from a pastiche of events, encounters, and friendships cultivated over the years. It is these experiences that led me to think seriously about the legacies of HIV interventions and the un/intended impacts of global health programs. Here I am reminded of James Ferguson's (1994) observation that development projects seem to fail with regular consistency. In his study of development in Lesotho, he urged us to reconsider how failure is not "doing nothing" but rather doing something else that "always has its own logic" (276). It is safe to say that most things fall into the gray areas between success and failure, intended and unintended, and it is the nebulous interplay of these spaces that forms the central inquiry of this book.

I begin by recounting the story of MSM testing in chapter 1, where I explore how and why MSM testing became the prevailing strategy to prevent and control the HIV epidemic in China. The embrace of this intervention, I show, came out of a concatenation of events, epidemiological and otherwise, that drew increased scrutiny to MSM and their roles in the sexual transmission of HIV. Here I introduce readers to ACF and the Health Fund, two key donors promoting this intervention in the country, and detail how each developed its respective MSM testing initiatives. Although the donors shared the same goal—to scale up testing among MSM in order to reduce transmission—their reasons for doing so arose out of very different motivations that shaped their MSM testing design and implementation decisions.

As MSM testing slowly rose in prominence in the public health landscape, donors and the community-based organizations tasked with scaling up MSM testing faced a challenge: how to mobilize MSM to get tested. I describe the response to this challenge in chapter 2. The construction of crisis around MSM produced an imagined population of "hidden" HIV-positive MSM "out there" within the general, heterosexual public. I show how making up MSM was pivotal to and at the same time shaped by MSM testing and the use of performance-based financing, thereby illustrating the productivity of testing as a technology. I pay special attention to practices of *ziworentong*, or self-affirmation, that reconfigured how Chinese men conceived of themselves and acted responsibly as MSM.

The making up of MSM became a crucial component to the success of scaling up testing among MSM as a public health strategy, as I detail in chapter 3. The popularity of testing eventually became integrated into the local public health systems in China, primarily through the practice of social service contracting or outsourcing HIV testing and other services to community-based organizations by the Chinese CDC. In this chapter, I examine how social service contracting organized around MSM testing has circumscribed the kinds of prevention and care available to MSM. By focusing primarily on testing and diagnosing MSM, but with few other forms of care included or acknowledged, this intervention has transformed MSM into commodities of care that accrue political and economic value—at times at the expense of their care.

The predominance of MSM testing gradually led to rifts and splinters within the community, that is, among activists and organizations providing HIV services to this population. I begin to explore the aftermath, or aftereffects, of this intervention as it unfolded across the communities (chapter 4) and lives (chapter 5) of MSM. A key question driving these two chapters is, what happens after testing? In chapter 4, I argue that this intervention and its effects have undermined the ability of community-based organizations and activists to advocate for MSM. Instead, the orientation toward testing MSM has unintentionally redefined the roles of organizations as service providers only, rather than as advocates for the communities they serve and, often, to which they belong. Here I show how organizations' involvement in testing has inadvertently limited their possibilities for broader forms of social engagement.

In chapter 5, I trace MSM testing in the lives of the men affected by this intervention. I share the stories of HIV-positive men and describe ways that they reconciled their newfound HIV status with the everyday realities and pressures of their lives. I show how many men responded to their HIV status by reimagining how to live as a "proper" HIV-positive Chinese MSM and how this conduct was variably interpreted and practiced by these men. By telling their stories, I underline yet again some of the gaps of MSM testing and the importance of situating technical interventions within the social worlds in which men live.

The lessons learned from MSM testing became apparent to me five years after I left the field, as I describe in the conclusion. I returned to China in 2015 to organize a workshop in Beijing as a follow-up to my research and found myself in the midst of animated and often heated debates about the effectiveness of MSM testing. I conclude by reflecting on how scaling up MSM testing, as part of broader trends in global health, has produced unexpected arrangements of governance and power along with unanticipated consequences for HIV prevention among MSM.

ONE

THE PRODUCTIVITY
OF HIV TESTING

IN SUMMER 2008, I arranged an interview with Thomas, a program officer with the Health Fund, an international organization dedicated to supporting health and development initiatives worldwide. At the time, I had only just started researching HIV in China, but already I was privy to the persistent rumors about the Health Fund's use of performance-based financing as a mechanism for scaling up HIV testing in "key populations" (e.g., sex workers, people who inject drugs, MSM). This mechanism involves tying monetary incentives to the delivery of performance targets or outputs by, for example, providing payments per HIV test administered or per person initiating antiretroviral therapy (ART). In the words of several critics I met, performance-based financing was, most simply, paying men to get tested. Intrigued by the mechanism and the controversy surrounding it, I was eager to speak to someone inside the organization to learn more. In July, that opportunity came by way of a friend and former consultant to the Health Fund, who put me in touch with Thomas, one of the program officers managing the Health Fund's HIV programs at the time.

The meeting started off as most of my meetings did: I introduced myself and my research interests and asked a set of questions about the organization's programs. I inquired about the Health Fund's goals and expectations, along with what it hoped to accomplish as a result of its program. At this point, the discussion turned to the Health Fund's monitoring and evaluation practices, now a mainstay of almost every global health and development initiative. Thomas explained that the primary objective of its HIV program was to bring down new infections in key populations, which at that time included sex workers, people who inject drugs, and MSM. Demonstrating results was an important part of the program design, according to Thomas, and a primary question driving the work was how well an intervention was doing what it was supposed to be doing.

To measure an intervention's effectiveness, the Health Fund established numerical outputs—for instance, how many HIV tests were administered, how many new HIV cases were identified, how many people initiated ART—for each population group. I asked if the assessment measures used were exclusively quantitative, to which Thomas replied, "Of course! How else do you measure effectiveness? How would you measure impact otherwise?" I speculated that any assessment tool used might depend on the kind of impact a program hoped to make because not all outcomes could be quantitatively measured. He agreed, and then explained, "It really depends on what kind of objective you develop at the beginning; effectiveness is measured by your outcomes against your original goals." To elaborate, Thomas pointed to the inadequacies of peer education, noting, "For example, I used to conduct peer-to-peer education, and everyone said, 'Oh, yes, this is really effective, and we've made real impacts,' but the rate of HIV infections had not gone down, and people were still contracting STIs. So, where was the impact?" In contrast, he emphasized, the uniqueness of the Health Fund program was that it incorporated concrete, quantitative targets that needed to be met by the end of the program to ensure its success. For this reason, only key populations were targeted, he explained:

> THOMAS: These groups are the main [HIV] carriers, so if you want to slow down the spread [of the epidemic], then you need to target these groups.
>
> ME: Isn't the HIV rate increasing as a result of heterosexual transmission?
>
> THOMAS: Of course, but who do you think these heterosexual groups are? How do you think they are contracting HIV if not in these [key population] groups? Here, let's pretend we have this cup of water, and that it is a high-risk group. Pick one.
>
> ME: How about female sex workers—
>
> THOMAS: OK, female sex workers. Now, the cup could overfill with water and then spread out to other members of society. But, if you could keep the water from overflowing, then you can prevent rising HIV rates. That's why you need prevention activities in

these communities, so that they can prevent the spread [of HIV].
If female sex workers could all use condoms during their activities,
then you could prevent the spread of HIV to other people.

His analogy, of course, could be extended to any key population,
and, indeed, that was the point. From the donor's perspective, population risk groups are interchangeable in this testing intervention so long
as they can be standardized. Thomas's reasoning as to how and why
these groups should be targeted presupposed yet also worked to flatten
the circumstances of HIV transmission in these groups, thereby disas-
sociating the epidemic from the social conditions that fuel it. Why certain groups had high or low HIV prevalence seemed to be less relevant
than treating all populations as the same for the purposes of measuring impact. The seductiveness of universalizing key populations like
MSM drives the push to scale up HIV testing in these groups, because
it shapes the kinds of data collected to allow for the comparison of results across multiple contexts.

* * * * *

Two years later, in 2010, I conducted a follow-up interview with Yang
Xia, the Health Fund program officer who took over Thomas's position
in managing the HIV portfolio, and with whom I worked closely during my time as a consultant, researcher, and volunteer with the Health
Fund. I was interested in hearing about how the program had pro-
gressed since my initial interview, when it had still been in the nascent
stages of implementation. By the time I returned to China for long-term
fieldwork, the program had been in operation for multiple years, giving the Health Fund time to work out any early kinks. In our meeting,
Yang Xia hit upon many of the same talking points as her predeces-
sor, highlighting the organization's focus on HIV testing, treatment,
and care among key populations. However, she pointed to one notable
change that had been made to the program. The Health Fund had reoriented the HIV testing component to MSM only and scaled back or
eliminated sex workers and people who inject drugs from this part of
the program.

I must have looked puzzled, because Yang Xia explained that this
decision had been made after data generated from the preliminary
stages of the program implementation showed few to no new HIV
cases identified in sex workers and people who inject drugs. As the

program rolled out gradually across the country, they consistently discovered few new HIV cases in these two populations. In some cities,
Yang Xia noted, zero HIV infections turned up. Their findings were
not altogether surprising, since, as she indicated, national statistics
demonstrated that HIV prevalence among sex workers was in decline.
Official reports at the time estimated HIV rates in this population to
be 0.6 percent and in people who inject drugs 9.3 percent (Ministry of
Health of the People's Republic of China [MHPRC] 2010). I asked what
she thought might account for the low numbers, and Yang Xia replied
that "in all likelihood . . . the same women in the same venues were
probably tested repeatedly," and they were perhaps not sex workers at
all, an occurrence other anthropologists have also described (see Hyde
2007; Mason 2016). Despite Yang Xia's acknowledgment that the data
were questionable, they were nonetheless accepted as "good enough"
(see Biruk 2018; Kaufman 2015) to convince the Health Fund to reduce
the resources it was investing in addressing HIV transmission among
these two populations.

In contrast, preliminary data related to MSM showed much higher
HIV infection rates than anticipated. Indeed, early data collected from
the Health Fund's program showed HIV incidence among MSM reaching upward of 10 percent in some cities, a finding that aligned with a
2008–9 national study that estimated that an average of 5 percent, but
in some urban centers greater than 10 percent, of all Chinese MSM
were HIV-positive (MHPRC, Joint UN Programme on HIV/AIDS,
and World Health Organization 2010). The Health Fund, drawing on
its and other data sources, decided to redirect its resources to scale
up HIV testing in MSM. In the words of Yang Xia, "We felt we were
spending a lot of money on these two groups [sex workers and people
who inject drugs] but with no results to show for it. We spent less
money on MSM yet yielded a lot more results. At the end of the day,
this is a results-based program and we need to see outcomes. We spent
all this money and it was simply inefficient; by refocusing our efforts on
MSM, the program will be much more financially efficient."

As we concluded our interview, Yang Xia, perhaps still sensing my
perplexity, reiterated the importance of measuring performance. As an
example, she criticized the Global Fund's activities in China, arguing
that "no one knows where the money goes." And that, it seemed, was
key. The Health Fund's programs, she countered, instituted clear tar-

gets across activities so as to ensure that its resources were used effi-
ciently, transparently, and in a cost-effective manner.

* * * * *

How did HIV testing in MSM become the prevailing strategy for
prevention and control in China? How did this intervention come to
govern, so to speak, the HIV landscape, reshaping the possibilities
for thinking about and acting upon the epidemic? And how did cost-
effectiveness, as emphasized by Yang Xia, come to guide decisions in
determining health priorities? The turn toward scaling up HIV testing
in MSM came out of a concatenation of events. HIV prevalence had
been rapidly rising, portending a potential crisis in this population.
This shift intersected temporally with an epidemiological change in
which sexual contact became the leading HIV transmission route in the
country in the mid-2000s. At the time of my fieldwork, sexual transmission accounted for 63.9 percent of existing HIV cases and 81.6 percent of new HIV infections; 17.4 percent of existing and 29.4 percent of
newly diagnosed infections were transmitted through homosexual contact (MHPRC 2012). Yet, what worried public health experts and HIV
activists was not transmission alone but the speed at which HIV infections were increasing in MSM. That many Chinese MSM are married
and live heterosexual lives further compounded these concerns and
reinforced an urgency to identify these men for the purposes of HIV
surveillance and prevention.

The epidemiological shifts in China emerged amid wider trends in
global health programs whereby donors increasingly demanded more
transparency and accountability in health spending. Concomitant with
these trends was an explosion and appropriation of business parlance
into health conversations: "return on investment," "cost-effectiveness,"
and "value for money" became central to health programming discourse.[1] This language shift reflected donors' embrace of business approaches to address health challenges. They aimed to maximize positive health impacts with each dollar spent. The gold standard in health
programs soon became a "statistically robust, randomized and controlled, cost-effectively constituted, experimentally designed, outcome-
measurable intervention/research project" (Adams 2016, 31)—one
that could be standardized, scaled up, and used comparatively across
multiple contexts. Marilyn Strathern (2000) has labeled this trend in

which accounting and accountability mechanisms drive institutional decisions, and in which we still find ourselves, an "audit regime." Yang Xia's criticism of the Global Fund's program for not knowing "where the money goes" reflects this new "audit culture."

In this chapter, I examine the rise of HIV testing among MSM as a key strategy in China, one that was intertwined with performance-based financing and other forms of incentivization. I also use this chapter to set the stage for understanding why making up MSM became crucial to this endeavor. HIV testing, I argue, is a versatile technology that does different things for different people and is not merely limited to its productivity as a technical intervention. It is as much a public health tool as it is an instrument of empowerment; yet, its implementation limits the possibilities by which HIV prevention is thinkable and actionable.

HIV INTERVENTIONS AND MSM

The Health Fund's prioritization of HIV testing among MSM was galvanized by two main drivers: the low HIV testing and detection rates in MSM when it began and the lack of robust metrics in existing HIV interventions. As Thomas and Yang Xia's comments revealed, there was a general dissatisfaction among international donors and leaders with the way health, especially HIV, programs had been administered in the past. The issue, expressed to me on several occasions by program staff, was that there was little accountability for how funding was distributed across HIV programs, and even less accounting of the impacts of programs intended to reduce HIV infections. As a consequence, low-performing programs that failed to demonstrate significant impacts and the organizations that administered them continued to receive funding.

Certainly, earlier HIV interventions in China looked significantly different than the performance-based models promulgated by the Health Fund. The initial phases of the HIV epidemic in the late 1980s and into the 1990s most directly affected people who inject drugs and sex workers, starting along the drug trafficking routes in southern China and spreading outward to nearby provinces. HIV responses at that time focused on strengthening national monitoring and surveillance systems under the guidance and support of international donors like WHO (Jia et al. 2007). As part of these efforts, national sentinel surveillance sites were rolled out across the country and key populations were integrated over time, allowing for better data collection and forecasting of epidemic trends. During this period, HIV interventions were primarily population specific. For instance, a combination of harm-reduction strategies, such as methadone-maintenance treatment and needle exchange programs, was expanded for people who inject drugs and later adopted into national policies after proving to be effective in slowing down the spread of HIV among this population (Cui, Liau, and Wu 2009). For sex workers, interventions such as condom promotion in entertainment venues, the establishment of STI clinics, and health education and counseling outreach activities enabled an increase in the rate of condom use and a decrease in the incidence of some STIs (Wu et al. 2007).

These endeavors signaled an important shift in the government's initially slow and even passive response to HIV, which had been widely criticized by international organizations (see UN Theme Group on HIV/AIDS in China 2002). Despite these laudatory efforts to take HIV seriously, the impacts of early programs were varied. For instance, in a report commissioned by the Center for Strategic and International Studies, authors indicated that most of the HIV interventions implemented in the 2000s were largely ineffective (Gill, Huang, and Lu 2007). As an example, they pointed to studies that countered the success of condom promotion strategies among sex workers, citing reports that showed that unprotected sex remained a common practice among sex workers.[2] Another study found that HIV rates increased among sex workers despite high rates of condom use in some regions (Lau et al. 2007).

Similar anthropological studies, including that of Shao-hua Liu (2010), which detailed the lives of heroin users in southwestern China, have described the failure of bilateral initiatives like the China–United Kingdom project to curb the spread of HIV among people who inject drugs. The success of needle exchange interventions touted in some studies had little positive impact in Shao-hua Liu's study site; instead, these efforts met with considerable resistance from community members and led to the criminalization of peer educators involved with the project. Liu attributed these failures partly to bureaucratic inadequacies and, as she put it, to cultural incompetence.

The mixed impacts of the HIV interventions I describe here pale, however, when compared to the virtual lack of data on the effectiveness of MSM-targeted programs in the 1990s and into the early 2000s. In part, this information deficit can be traced to the limited surveillance of the MSM population, which marginalized MSM from the HIV response. Unlike the immediate incorporation of sex workers and people who inject drugs into sentinel surveillance systems in 1995, MSM were only added in 2003 and, even then, were not included at every site (He and Detels 2005). No doubt the pathologization of same-sex sexual practices and early denial of its existence in the country contributed to this absence. The result was an overrepresentation of certain populations in HIV surveillance to the detriment of harder-to-reach groups like MSM (Gill, Huang, and Lu 2007; Kaufman, Kleinman, and Saich 2006; Zhang et al. 2012). This underrepresentation not only rendered MSM marginal, if not invisible, to HIV interventions but also ensured that few resources were being directed their way.

Owing to the limited data available about MSM, there was little governmental effort to seriously address HIV prevention in this population prior to the Health Fund. Instead, interventions were sporadic and piecemeal, reflecting the sparse yet slowly emerging data. The earliest initiatives targeting MSM primarily focused on providing HIV-related information and support by way of telephone hotlines, digital and mass media, and venue-based services, carried out by a handful of academic and community-based organizations (Kaufman 2011). These interventions were implemented in response to data that showed that a key barrier to MSM participating in HIV prevention programs was the low perception of HIV risk by MSM, even as they engaged in sexual practices that put them at risk for infection (Choi et al. 2002; Choi et al. 2004; Zhang et al. 2000). For example, public health studies pointed to the multiple number of sexual partners and high rates of unprotected sex among MSM, practices exacerbated by the strong social expectations for Chinese men to get married and establish families (Choi et al. 2002; Zhang and Chu 2005). This information, combined with the limited surveillance of MSM, led some to speculate that the actual number of HIV-positive MSM far exceeded the projected estimates (Gill, Huang, and Lu 2007).

The low HIV risk perception among MSM may also account, at least in part, for the low HIV testing rates in the population, which was compounded by the number of men not aware of their HIV status. It should be noted that HIV testing rates in general and not just among MSM have been low, historically, in China (Wu, Rou, and Cui 2004). However, among MSM, they were alarmingly so; one study reported that 18 percent of the men in their surveys had ever been tested for HIV, and of those who tested HIV-positive, 93 percent did not know their status prior to getting tested (Choi et al. 2006). The nature of these findings have since been corroborated by additional research (Fan et al. 2012; He et al. 2006; Wei et al. 2014).[3] Later interventions, therefore, scaled up existing activities and added condom promotion, counseling and testing, HIV and STI services, theme parties, and peer and internet-based education in a bid to widen the scale and scope of MSM-targeted interventions (Cui, Liau, and Wu 2009; Sun et al. 2010).

By the mid-2000s, MSM began to garner more attention in the national HIV response. For example, they were included, during multiple Global Fund grant cycles, as a key population to be targeted for HIV prevention. These grants largely supported community-based organizations to carry out interventions, and over the years, MSM groups have received a bulk of Global Fund money (Huang and Jia 2014). In turn, the number of MSM organizations proliferated (Li et al. 2010). Despite the increased attention given to MSM, however, there were few substantive data on the impact or effectiveness of the new and growing number of interventions, at least, prior to the arrival of the Health Fund.

The Global Fund offers an illustrative example for making sense of the Health Fund's grievance regarding the accountability of existing HIV interventions, especially those targeting MSM. In a study of the Global Fund's HIV/AIDS programs in China, Huang Yanzhong and Jia Ping (2014) pointed to the consistently low value for money resulting from their grants, meaning they were not maximizing the benefits from each dollar spent in their projects. The authors suggest that the increased resources directed to MSM groups have done little to curb HIV infections in this population, an observation supported by a report published in 2013 showing a rise in HIV prevalence among MSM, despite an increase of consistent condom use and an uptick in HIV testing (Lu et al. 2013). The problem of low value for money has been exacerbated by the persistent misuse of funding by government institutions and the lack of built-in accountability metrics that allow for the monitoring of health spending and health impact, according to many staff members at the Health Fund. This issue had partly to do with the way international projects, including the Health Fund's, are filtered through national and local government channels in China. In the case of HIV, that channel was the Chinese CDC. Even though the Global Fund was one of the earliest institutions to embrace and promote performance metrics in order to maximize value for money in its programs, the way its projects unfolded in the Chinese context did not always align with its expectations. Similarly, how the Health Fund's HIV program played out, as will become evident throughout this book, incidentally provides an apt example of this disconnect. As Huang and Jia explained, the emphasis on value for money generates incentives for grant recipients to report positive results, even when programs have little impact on the ground.

It is against this backdrop that the Health Fund arrived in China.

HIV TESTING AND PAYMENT FOR PERFORMANCE

The Health Fund's HIV program had, at its core, a public health goal: to reduce and control new HIV infections. To do this, the organization adopted a test and treat strategy into its HIV program, which promoted initiating ART immediately upon an HIV diagnosis regardless of CD4 count so as to reduce viral loads in persons and thereby lessen the likelihood of passing the virus to others.[4] This model gained considerable traction globally during the 2000s and has been advocated by public health scholars as an effective, and cost-effective, method to decrease HIV transmission in a population (Dieffenbach and Fauci 2009; Gilks et al. 2006; Granich et al. 2009; Montaner et al. 2006).[5]

At the time of the Health Fund's arrival in China in the 2000s, HIV testing did not yet command serious attention as a prevention strategy, much less as a strategy to be used among MSM (though a handful of studies indicated potential utility; see Choi et al. 2004; Choi et al. 2006). Earlier efforts to expand voluntary counseling and testing (VCT) services in the country failed to demonstrate much utilization of these services even after the government made HIV testing free at all health facilities. HIV testing generated more interest after a 2004 and 2005 national effort to actively test key populations identified a larger than expected number of HIV-positive persons and allowed the government to minimize the gap between estimated and confirmed HIV cases (Gill, Huang, and Lu 2007). Even then, however, interest in testing remained limited to members of public health communities. The campaign at this time—described as an opt-out campaign because individuals were tested unless they opted out—was controversial in nature and limited in reach, because active testing was only done in venues like detox and detention centers, in STI clinics that catered to sex workers and people who inject drugs, and in geographically concentrated areas to test rural persons who contracted HIV from commercial blood and plasma stations (Wu et al. 2006). MSM, however, were not yet being consistently reached.

The adoption of HIV testing among MSM by the Health Fund helped create critical inroads for shifting national attention, and resources, to MSM. Testing promised to remedy many of the shortfalls that plagued earlier interventions because it had the capacity to diagnose and to measure. The rationale behind this strategy, Yang Xia explained, was that if a person is aware of his HIV status, then he will presumably adjust his sexual practices accordingly or initiate and maintain ART so he is less likely to transmit the virus to others. There is also another utility to this intervention: HIV tests are things, objects, that are countable and hence amenable to the kinds of accountability metrics the Health Fund desired.

Indeed, the need for governance and accountability underpinned the design and implementation of the Health Fund's HIV program. As Yann, the director of the Health Fund at the time, explained to me, "in the past, traditional donor/grantee relationships had a lot less accountability and transparency in the use of funding." He advocated, instead, for moving into a fee-for-service type of arrangement by which payments are rendered in relation to performance—that is, paid upon the delivery of services. This way, he reasoned, grantees will "only get paid based on what they produce; they must show outputs, rather than taking the money and then using it and reporting back. This makes it much more difficult to cheat," a suspicion that prevailed among many donors and stakeholders with whom I interacted in the field. To Yann, the need to adopt alternative health models came down to accountability. As he explained, "under older models of aid, these groups could get away with less work for the same amount of money," because payments were provided in advance. The old structure left donors with little oversight of quality control.

It seemed apt, then, that the Health Fund incorporated performance-based financing (or performance incentives) into its HIV program, building considerations of cost management into the program design. Defined as the "transfer of money or material goods conditional on taking a measurable action or achieving a predetermined performance target" (Eichler, Levine, and the Performance-Based Incentives Working Group [PBI] 2009, 6), performance-based financing ties payments to performance targets or outputs like the number of vaccinations administered, the number of patients treated by a given institution, or the achievement of results. Donors usually favor this method because it provides them the kind of measurable impacts that carry purchase in global health programs, and it facilitates accountability for spending. In other words, with performance-based financing, "you get what you pay for. And it is easier to pay for what you can easily measure" (Eichler, Levine, and PBI 2009, 42).

These kinds of incentives have been promoted for decades as a way to achieve important, and calculable, health gains. The mechanism is not about "reducing costs or cutting budgets, but rather about maximizing the health impact of every available peso, pound, or pula to reduce human suffering and save lives. Or, simply put, getting more health for the money" (Glassman, Fan, and Over 2013, ix). Performance-based financing, and similar kinds of metrics, become especially important in times of financial exigency or in resource-limited settings. Consider, for example, quality-adjusted life year (QALY) and disability-adjusted life year (DALY), which were utilized by the World Bank in the 1990s to address concerns about how to measure health in terms of cost. QALY, argued Vincanne Adams (2016, 27), emerged out of a "crisis of *funding*" that motivated the Global North to calculate the cost of keeping people alive, while DALY arose during a "crisis of *data*" that justified continued investments for diseases in the Global South. These metrics helped to facilitate comparisons of disease and other conditions across contexts and guided donors' decision-making in setting health priorities. Undoubtedly, the history and reported success of these earlier mechanisms shaped the Health Fund's decision to divert its resources away from sex workers and people who inject drugs and toward MSM.

In practice, Health Fund staff had minimal oversight of the actual carrying out of HIV testing, given that everyday financing and program management came under the purview of government intermediaries. Although this structure was partly out of necessity, it was also by design: metrics-driven programs standardize targets and payments, thereby enabling donors to take a more "hands-off" approach. In theory, what mattered more than how the targets were met was whether they were met at all, and the cost for doing so. However, as I discuss later in this chapter, the use of performance-based financing did not roll out quite as expected in the Chinese context.

* * * * *

The Health Fund staff envisioned its HIV program to be "pioneering" for bringing alternative models and approaches to HIV prevention in China. As Yann articulated in an international health conference organized in Beijing, a key goal of the Health Fund was to ensure that interventions actually work as intended and can demonstrate measurable impact. The organization's foray into China signaled a different way of "doing" health, so to speak—one that prioritized a "Money, Markets, Measurement, and Management" approach and privileged the delivery of economic and scientific metrics (Ramdas 2011, 394).

A key part of the Health Fund's HIV program involved developing appropriate metrics for holding grantees accountable and measuring the impacts of interventions. Their program, in principle, advanced a comprehensive approach to HIV prevention, starting from the initial HIV screening to posttest care and support.[6] HIV testing had been outsourced to community-based organizations, premised on the notion not only that these groups were more likely to access MSM but that men were more inclined to go to them for HIV services, given the stigmatization they often experienced at government-run facilities (Feng, Wu, and Detels 2010). The role of these community-based organizations extended to recruiting and referring MSM to government public health facilities (VCTs, the Chinese CDC) for testing, pre- and posttest counseling, and monitoring of treatment adherence, as needed.

To obtain funding, grantee organizations submitted proposals to their local government intermediaries detailing the number of MSM they anticipated reaching per project period, along with other numerical targets. These targets were then measured against the actual number of men reached as verified by the Chinese CDC, because all testing and confirmation of an HIV diagnosis must go through the government to be eligible for free ART. If a person was confirmed to be HIV-positive by the Chinese CDC, then his personal information (such as name, contact information, and identity card [shenfenzheng]) would be uploaded into a national database to allow for regular monitoring of his progress.[7] Payments to community-based organizations, in turn, were allocated based on performance incentives set by the Health Fund, calculated at a fixed amount per MSM referred to HIV testing and an additional monetary reward per HIV-positive result. Thus, while an organization might have requested CNY 5,000 (USD 726) to reach a hundred MSM for HIV testing, for example, at the end of the project period, that organization may only have received CNY 2,500 (USD 363) if it was only able to mobilize fifty men. Add to this the fact that any person who was confirmed to be HIV-positive yielded the grantee organization an additional monetary incentive that amounted to at least five times more than that provided for an HIV test.[8] As a result, how well an organization performed in reaching its estimated target was an important factor in determining the organization's future financial viability.

The Health Fund counted things differently and counted different things than the Global Fund. In the latter's programs, for instance, organizations applied for funding based on the completion of activities, such as the number of workshops organized or the number of informational materials or condoms distributed. As Thomas asked at the start of this chapter, however, "how do you measure effectiveness"—in this case, specifically, of an activity like a workshop? In contrast to the Global Fund, the Health Fund staff counted outputs in the form of the number of men receiving an HIV test, the number of men testing positive for HIV, and the number of men initiating ART, among other things, to demonstrate calculable impacts. By utilizing this method of counting, they were able to show cost-effectiveness in terms of the unit cost per HIV case detected and impact in terms of the number of HIV cases identified as well as the number of men who initiated ART.

The generalizability of the Health Fund's intervention was of crucial importance to Health Fund staff. As Yang Xia explained to me, they had hopes of replicating and exporting this HIV testing model in China to other HIV-affected areas of the world. Yet, at the time of my fieldwork, she confided that "right now, there is no evidence that our model . . . is any more effective than what is already being done." This lack of data posed a problem, because "our models must be evidence based; it is about presenting the numbers to prove our model works, or that it is at least cost-effective." Without sufficient numbers, the program office in China risked being unable to convince its administrators at the international level to keep the program going. In contrast, if it could prove the model worked, it could export it globally. The intended portability of this intervention intensified the need to generate numbers, and "good" numbers, as evidence of the model's effectiveness.

The privileging of portability is a residual effect of evidence-based medicine (EBM) and its incursion into public health. Introduced in the 1990s, EBM gradually became institutionalized across health sectors to guide medical care and, at the same time, authorize the scientific validity of numbers and statistics as the best kind of evidence with which to make clinical decisions. It is predicated on standardization across all aspects of medical care, creating a kind of internal consistency that requires treating all patients as interchangeable to measure the efficacy of medical practices (Timmermans and Mauck 2005; see also Bell 2017). In global health, EBM encouraged precisely the kinds of interventions the Health Fund embraced, interventions that demonstrated tangible, evidence-based results and could travel across diverse contexts. MSM as a key population mattered to the Health Fund so long as they continued to generate good numbers to justify continued investments into their community. It becomes worth asking in such a context, what happens to these men when the numbers no longer justify the investments?

PERFORMING FOR PAYMENT

The pressure to generate numbers and meet targets in the Health Fund's program unexpectedly led to a series of incidents that threatened to undermine the enterprise of HIV testing in MSM as an effective prevention strategy. From the outset, the HIV program was beset with counting problems—that is, who got counted in HIV testing and how people were counted. The solution to these problems, it seemed, was to enhance accountability measures used to monitor funding, which took the form of increased paperwork, adding layers of bureaucratic oversight to community-based organizations and government intermediaries. Still, that such issues arose exposes the unintended consequences of portable interventions when they collide with local contexts and practices that disrupt their seamless transfer from one point to the next. Such disruptions, I quickly discovered, translated into an array of questionable practices by multiple stakeholders as they sought to navigate an expanding field of metrics that simultaneously narrowed the purview of HIV prevention in China. HIV testing inevitably morphed into an intervention not to save lives per se but rather to test as many men as possible.

I had long heard rumors of deception, or "cheating," in the Health Fund's program even before I got involved, and the stories continued to abound well into my time there. I recall, for instance, a meeting I once attended with Health Fund staff and government intermediaries in which the participants complained about the problem of "repeat testers," that is, persons who were referred to multiple locations by a grantee organization to get tested for HIV. This had become a relatively widespread practice, deployed as a way for organizations to accumulate additional incentives, because organizations received monetary rewards per person getting tested. Furthermore, a person could be counted multiple times toward an organization's estimated targets. According to some government staff, this deception could be attributed to the low incentive given per HIV test; as one government official stated, "there is no motivation for MSM groups to go out and do outreach because the payment for an HIV test is not enough."

The Health Fund staff were well aware of these problems, as indicated in the meeting I described earlier, among many others I attended. And the issue of "repeat testers" was not the only dilemma to arise. I regularly encountered stories of non-MSM getting referred to public health institutions to get tested and counted so that community-based organizations could meet performance targets and collect incentives. Zhang Li, with whom I worked closely at ACF, but who also consulted on the Health Fund's HIV program, confirmed as much to me: "in some places, community-based organizations will go out and mobilize migrant laborers that are not MSM to get tested; they did so by sharing the performance incentive with the laborer getting tested." This arrangement of splitting incentives became a growing practice among many community-based organizations involved in the Health Fund program. I recall one incident that occurred during a trip I took with staff from the Health Fund to a program site. During a conversation I had with a volunteer from a grantee organization, the volunteer described to me how his organization split the incentive with the men getting tested, giving half the amount to the men and keeping the remainder for themselves, unbeknownst to the Health Fund program officer with us at the time. Because of the speed at which this practice spread, the Health Fund had to explicitly ban the arrangement.

A more pernicious rumor I came across while in the field involved collusion between public health institutions (such as the Chinese CDC) and community-based organizations to fabricate data in order to collect and share performance incentives. In at least one instance, an organization involved with both ACF's Test, Treat, and Prevent project and with the Health Fund's program revealed that it had arranged to split the performance incentives with its local CDC branch so long as the organization brought men getting tested for HIV to its specific office rather than another CDC branch. Still more serious allegations concerned local CDC offices manipulating data regarding the number of HIV-positive cases identified by a community-based organization to claim the higher incentives given for new HIV cases, given that all HIV cases need to be verified by the CDC.

To be clear, I did not personally witness any such acts of deception during my time in the field; however, these stories were a part of nearly every meeting I attended at the Health Fund, as staff struggled to develop new ways of ensuring accountability. These stories circulated across the HIV landscape as a "public secret" (Geissler 2013) and worked to reinforce the perception that accountability metrics like performance-based financing were necessary. Of course, data manipulation has been a long-standing problem in China, as other scholars have shown (Liu 2010; Mason 2016). The problems experienced by the Health Fund were not isolated but part of a broader social and cultural landscape in which scientific data circulate as political capital.

The challenges besieging the Health Fund were characteristic of many international projects in the country. Here again, the Global Fund offers an exemplary case study. In 2010–11, at the time of my research, the Global Fund suspended and later froze its grants to China, citing financial mismanagement and the failure of the government to properly distribute funding to community-based organizations. This abuse can be blamed partly on the decentralized nature of the public health system that subjects local CDC offices to the administrative leadership of their territorial governments (Huang and Jia 2014). This structure meant that local governments had a vested interest in keeping the money in their systems in the form of subsidies rather than passing it on to organizations as stipulated in the grant. Furthermore, given how fragmented government branches are in the country, a lack of coordination made transparency in spending impossible, a consequence that Shao-hua Liu (2010) also found in the China–United Kingdom project in the Southwest.

Various forms of financial mismanagement can be said to have evolved out of the marketization of health care in the country. Deng Xiaoping's ushering in of privatization and decentralization in the late 1970s led to significant reductions in central government provision of health financing. Instead, health facilities had to seek out alternative ways to sustain their operations independently, leading many to turn to fee-for-service models to generate income. Public health systems faced similar challenges, as the ability of local governments to maintain health care facilities depended on local financial conditions. The outcome of such processes over time, as Liu (2010) showed, was that health workers came to see public health work as a burden. In Liu's words, "the state can no longer expect health workers to do as much as they used to if the state does not appropriately reward them with tangible benefits" (140).

The adoption of performance-based financing, then, did not cause deception, but it did introduce new ways for such existing practices to manifest—and evolve. There are three points to which I want to draw attention here that are vital to understanding acts of duplicity in the context of testing MSM. First, the importance of getting "good data" for community-based organizations and donors alike is as valuable as attaining a positive health result (Adams 2013, 68). After all, consistently meeting one's estimated targets translates into financial viability and sustainability for community-based organizations. These considerations were especially salient given that international donors, once a bulwark of HIV support, had dwindled at the time of my fieldwork, thus increasing competition for what little funding remained. Relatedly, for donors like the Health Fund, good data serve as evidence of the effectiveness of their interventions. Second, the alleged inclusion of migrant laborers who are not MSM raises questions about who is counted in HIV testing. It also underlines the necessity of making up MSM, as I discuss in the next chapter, to meet HIV testing targets in donor programs. The "capaciousness" (Biruk 2019) of MSM as a category is key to this endeavor, because it allows for a diversity of men to be counted as performance targets and incentives, rather than only focusing on men claiming a particular identity. And third, community-based organizations and government institutions alike are learning how to perform accountability to access resources of care, rather than learning how to care (McKay 2018, 78; see also Sullivan 2017). As Zhang Li explained to me once, "these [subversive] practices happened because grantees learned over time how to fill out paperwork and gather receipts rather than do the work." In her estimation, had donors simply trusted organizations, instead of imposing ever-more accountability measures, duplicity may never have become an issue.

HIV TESTING AS AN INSTRUMENT OF EMPOWERMENT

Shortly after the Health Fund's HIV program started, ACF developed its own HIV testing initiative, Test, Treat, and Prevent, partly as a palliative to the Health Fund's program, even though it did so with a generous grant from the Health Fund to support the project. Jonah, the director of ACF, had been well aware of the many challenges surrounding the Health Fund's program and therefore designed this project to achieve the same HIV testing goals, this time, however, by reinforcing the centrality of care. He often compared the success of ACF's project to the failure of the Health Fund's programs when it came not only to generating good numbers but, more importantly, to cultivating trust. For Jonah, HIV testing did not just hold epidemiological promise; it became a tool of empowerment for MSM.

Jonah first began thinking about HIV testing in the late 2000s, after the Health Fund's program was already in place. At that time, ACF had not yet shifted into direct project implementation but rather still functioned as a grant maker, administering seed grants to community-based organizations to provide support to people living with HIV, including but not limited to MSM. The idea for HIV testing of MSM really emerged out of a series of conversations Jonah had been having with grassroots activists who, for years, had tried to bring attention to the growing epidemic in MSM. These activists were increasingly frustrated by what they saw to be the adverse effects of donors pushing performance metrics and paperwork that did little to stem HIV infections in their communities. They blamed these donor programs for the proliferation of "fake" organizations that took up HIV resources but did little work. These activists were among the first to distrust the numbers reported by such programs, and yet they did not know how to obtain more accurate (in their perception) data about HIV rates among MSM.

In short, they felt stymied in their attempts to push for HIV testing outside of existing structures.

This sense of powerlessness, Jonah claimed, was the genesis for the Test, Treat, and Prevent project. Indeed, ACF staff and, especially, Jonah were guided by strong commitments to mobilizing a grassroots movement to address HIV, and over the years, the organization expanded its programmatic repertoire to focus foremost on capacity building among community-based and grassroots organizations. This new initiative aligned perfectly with its mission. Jonah immediately began looking into rapid HIV testing as something local organizations could administer directly, thereby giving men an alternative to government public health institutions for testing. He drew on international best practices that placed a strong emphasis on pre- and post-test counseling as a mechanism of support, instead of adopting what he perceived to be a more clinical approach whereby HIV testing was administered as a clinical act (e.g., the extraction of blood) carried out in hospitals and other medical facilities in China. Instead, he envisioned a social world in which testing could be carried out by and for MSM throughout an array of gay-friendly spaces, including bars and bathhouses. To this end, Jonah eschewed the standard questionnaires used by the Chinese CDC and designed his own, asking fewer questions about men's sexual history and more about their testing habits. He also located a manufacturing company in the country that could produce rapid HIV testing kits at an affordable price and partnered with an international organization to train staff and volunteers in local organizations to carry out rapid HIV testing.

From its inception, ACF's Test, Treat, and Prevent project had as its goal the empowerment of individuals and communities to take control of their health. As Jonah explained, "I wanted quality testing, not quantity testing." For this reason, ACF's project did not require organizations to meet specific targets, although it did require grantees to report their testing numbers. Jonah attributed the (at least perceived) absence of duplicity among grantee organizations to this measure of reporting, not fulfilling. He surmised that "because I did not demand numbers from them, they felt more committed to testing and caring for MSM, rather than just collecting tests for the sake of meeting targets and getting incentives." For ACF, it was not about the numbers but rather about follow-up. Jonah asked of his grantees, "Can you follow up with the men you test, can you support them through the entire process if the men are HIV-positive?" Just like the Health Fund, ACF counted different things and counted things differently. The what and how in these two cases, importantly, were not the same.

One of the questions ACF staff asked on the pretest questionnaire was whether the person had ever been tested before. ACF staff quickly learned that most of the men coming into community-based organizations for HIV testing were first-time testers, indicating a need to expand outreach but also to innovate different kinds of support for this population to move beyond simply testing. One result was a complementary focus on promoting self-acceptance as a same-sex desiring man in the *ziworentong* project (see the next chapter).

Jonah had pride in ACF's project as being distinct from other existing projects that emphasized testing MSM (e.g., the Health Fund). Instead of providing performance incentives as other donors did, ACF opted to give in-kind support to its grantees, paying for direct costs like rapid HIV testing kits, travel, and accommodation to attend quarterly trainings; regular teleconferencing between grantee organizations; and allowances for modest stipends to support outreach activities.

In addition to these material benefits, a key component of ACF's project was accompaniment—that is, volunteers were required to follow up consistently with men who tested HIV-positive for a minimum of one month after the testing process. Forms of support included escorting men to the Chinese CDC for confirmation testing or CD4 testing to determine one's eligibility for ART; assisting with procuring ART, as needed; referring men to additional counseling and care services; and providing personalized support via talk and text. ACF, in Jonah's estimation, prioritized caring for men beyond getting them tested for HIV. For him, this aspect served not only to reduce the loss to follow-up rate (the proportion of men lost after an HIV screening) (see Chow, Wilson, and Zhang 2012) but also to build a sense of community for the men.

The accompaniment component of ACF's Test, Treat, and Prevent project was not the only innovative feature of the project, according to Jonah. ACF also utilized rapid HIV tests, which offer a quicker turnaround (generally within thirty minutes) than conventional methods (such as ELISA or western blot), in which the clinical extraction of blood is sent to a laboratory for testing and results can take days or weeks to return. Instead, rapid HIV tests use a retractable needle that delivers a quick prick to the finger to elicit small drops of blood and therefore can be administered by nonmedical professionals in nonlaboratory settings. This method, particularly when utilized by community-based organizations, offers MSM an alternative to getting tested at government-run facilities or fee-based hospitals, where experiences of stigmatization and breaches of confidentiality are often cited as reasons for low testing rates (Huang et al. 2012; Tao et al. 2014; Wei et al. 2014).

Despite their goals to build community among MSM, ACF's project did receive its fair share of critics, who accused Jonah of damaging the community. Many HIV activists criticized Jonah's acceptance of Health Fund money, accusing Jonah of siphoning away money from local Chinese organizations.[9] As one activist complained to me, "the Health Fund's program is already ruining the community . . . no grassroots group gets any of the money" and blamed ACF's project for having the same effect. Jonah downplayed such attacks, stating that at the end of the day, the money still went to community-based organizations. Instead, he praised Yann, director of the Health Fund, for "taking a risk with this project" by investing in ACF's Test, Treat, and Prevent project, because in the end, the project offered more than simply testing services. "Testing is not just a tool," Jonah once told me. "It is a human right [renquan]." Jonah envisioned HIV testing as a way for men to take control of their sexual health and desires to pursue same-sex relations. In his understanding, HIV testing empowered men to recognize and act on their same-sex desires as MSM, and to do so safely and responsibly.

MSM AS CARE, COMMUNITY, AND COMMODITY

An important part of ACF's project, specifically designed to build empowerment, was the quarterly workshop, organized every three months for three days. These workshops were designed to provide a space for sharing, learning, and networking among grantee organizations, and they incorporated a variety of subjects, ranging from the pragmatic, such as learning how to safely administer rapid HIV testing, to the conceptual, like understanding why attendees were doing HIV testing of MSM at all. It was through these workshops that fostering community became possible. Indeed, as Vinh-Kim Nguyen (2010, 58) observed, workshops do not simply translate institutional practices into local interventions; they act as transformative spaces, "fashioning selves and through them new kinds of social relations."

Each of the quarterly workshops followed a script, even as the topics varied. Jonah, as the facilitator, set the tone by establishing the ground rules on the first day, underlining the importance of listening and learning rather than judging. He insisted on making participants understand their role in the wider HIV testing apparatus—not as saviors but as interlocutors. "There is no savior syndrome allowed," he declared. "No one is here to save the world." Instead, he encouraged participants to share their experiences—successes and failures alike—with each other, acknowledging that the discussions were not meant to produce consensus but rather to reaffirm the commitments of those present to HIV testing and MSM. Unlike the typical lecture-dense sessions characteristic of Chinese conferences, these three-day workshops were filled with role-playing exercises, group activities, and peer-to-peer training, intended to foster interaction and participation.

Invariably, the workshops opened with a discussion about the need for rapid HIV testing in MSM. This was done partly to ensure that participants had a clear understanding of the project goals but also to gauge their commitment to the process. Jonah repeatedly stated that the aim of Test, Treat, and Prevent was not to deliver numbers but to deliver care to MSM. Therefore he initiated these conversations by asking participants to share their personal motivations for joining the project.

In most of the workshops I attended, community was a recurring theme. For example, I recall participants pointing out that MSM felt more comfortable going to them for HIV testing than getting tested at government health facilities, especially the Chinese CDC. As one man explained, "a *nantong* [man attracted to other men] coming in for an HIV test is more at ease with another *nantong* administering the test because he feels less judged." Another participant echoed this sentiment, sharing the following story:

> A client [*kehu*] came to us because he wanted to get tested for HIV since he had been having sex with men. He didn't want his wife to know why he needed to get tested. He had gone to the Chinese CDC but didn't like their attitude and didn't trust them to protect his confidentiality, so he came to us instead. I spent a lot of time talking to him and comforting him, and eventually we were able to work it

out and get him tested. Our services can help people like this man, who was so agitated initially but managed to come to terms with his situation.

In response to this, one participant remarked, "It is the community helping itself" *(ziji bang ziji)*. Jonah clearly agreed, exclaiming,

> Precisely! This is why, in our project we do not chase numbers. . . .
> Our project is like taking a car in for regular maintenance to ensure that there will be no problems, whereas other projects take the car in for maintenance only when there is a problem. . . . But if you bought a car, you would be attentive to it, taking it in regularly for repairs to make sure it is in good working condition.

HIV testing should not be undertaken only as a preventative precaution, Jonah meant; it should be integrated into one's lifestyle.

Here again, we see the emphasis not only on care but on the quality of that care exhibited in ACF's projects. Jonah was clear to distinguish between testing as a clinical act for the purpose of HIV surveillance and testing as an act of care, of the self and of others. He configured the act of testing as a form of care that is inseparable from the delivery of care as a deeply relational endeavor. That is to say, how HIV testing is delivered mattered—to Jonah, and to the workshop attendees who spoke out—as much as if not more so than who was delivering care. The "who" perhaps articulates most effectively the distinction between testing as a clinical act—provided by an anonymous medical professional—and testing as care by a peer, another MSM with whom one has a deeper affinity. Jonah insisted that care should not mean administering an HIV test only; instead, it should be part of a wider regimen of support that attends to the physical, emotional, and social health of a person, all delivered as part of a humanitarian ethos and community effort to save lives *(jiuming)*. For this reason, it seemed all the more salient that care be delivered to MSM and by MSM, according to Jonah and the workshop participants.

Jonah suggested that the absence of such care accounted for the reporting of inaccurate numbers in other testing initiatives like that of the Health Fund. Indeed, many participants acknowledged the pressure they felt to continually produce numbers in these programs. In one instance, the director of a community-based organization involved with ACF and the Health Fund's initiatives admitted to me that he submitted the same report with the same numbers three years in a row to the Health Fund, exhausted by the pressure to perform and the sheer amount of paperwork required. Yet, in admitting to me his indiscretion, he also expressed a dismissal of the importance of these numbers in relation to the humanitarian purpose for getting men tested. This sentiment undergirded the uniqueness of ACF's project, as a participant once noted: "this one [project] is good because we don't feel the pressure of needing to carry out testing; it is more about the follow-up activities after the testing."

Jonah encouraged participants to stay focused on care as the marker of their success: "You should not be concerned with finding the highest number of HIV-positive men or thinking that you need to have the right numbers to be successful." And yet, he stopped short of discounting the salience of numbers altogether, because, he admitted, it was ACF's numbers that got it the Health Fund's grant in the first place. Certainly, ACF also collected numbers from its grantee organizations, asking grantees to report their results. He reframed the purpose of generating numbers as ancillary to the greater goal of HIV care but not as something to be dismissed outright. Jonah made it clear to participants that, so long as the numbers provided to ACF were accurate, he did not mind if these same numbers were used elsewhere, for example, reported to the Health Fund to collect performance incentives, saying, "even if the number [of new HIV cases] for ACF is zero, then I do not care if you use these numbers to submit to other HIV testing projects to collect on performance incentives."

Jonah both critiqued number chasing and remained cognizant of the financial challenges of ACF's grantees, challenges that could be mitigated by the numbers. As an alternative to number chasing, Jonah pushed the groups to consider charging modest fees for their rapid HIV testing services. This became a topic of vociferous debate, as I witnessed at one of the workshops I attended in 2011, where participants argued for and against the merits of this practice. Representatives of a few of the grantee organizations worried that charging might discourage men from coming to them for HIV testing altogether. One participant asked, "Where is our comparative advantage if VCT centers and the Chinese CDC all offer testing for free?" Others questioned whether their work could still be considered charity if they were paid for their services.

Jonah actively advocated for charging fees, if only to promote the long-term sustainability of the community-based organizations. He asked some of the participants who had taken up this practice to share their experiences with the larger group. In response, the director of a group from central China described how the group recently started to charge CNY 20 (USD 3) per rapid HIV test. He explained that the organization had found that most of the men who came in were more than willing to pay that amount when they learned of all that the service entailed. In effect, the customers decided the service had good value for their money.

By encouraging a market-oriented approach to HIV testing, Jonah attended to organizations' financial sustainability, effectively suturing financial goals to the social goals of HIV prevention. His rationale was not unlike that of the leaders and staff of the Health Fund. He, too, linked health outcomes to financial outcomes while ensuring value for money. These logics reaffirmed an oft-made argument by philanthrocapitalists—a term coined to describe the emulation of for-profit practices to philanthropic endeavors—that economic pursuits need not be antithetical to social goals (Bishop and Green 2008).[10]

Philanthrocapitalist inklings have undoubtedly shaped testing MSM for HIV in China, whether by motivating the use of performance incentives or the practice of charging nominal fees for HIV testing. Economic self-interest, philanthrocapitalist logics suggest, no longer needs to be masked or minimized but should be leveraged as an effective way to help others, as Linsey McGoey (2016, 20; see also Birn 2014) has critiqued. The pursuit of economic interests, as a result, has played a powerful role in structuring HIV interventions in China, making possible new kinds of social value, social ties, and social networks (Elyachar 2005) that are now critical to preventing HIV in MSM. Yet, these principles coincide with a new development taking place: the making up of MSM, a practice by which philanthrocapitalist endeavors to address HIV in China were made possible.

CONCLUSION

In this chapter, I have examined the rise of HIV testing among MSM as a key strategy to prevent and control the epidemic in China, exploring both its utility as a technical intervention and its versatility as an instrument of care. Testing had already risen to predominance in the

HIV landscape by the time I arrived for fieldwork, and the Health Fund and ACF were two major players pushing forward this initiative. As I described, the motivations underpinning these two initiatives were starkly different, in ways that shaped the design and implementation of MSM testing but also the meaning behind testing itself. The Health Fund's testing initiative was informed by the demand for accounting and accountability of their funding, partly in response to a distrust of, or at least misgivings about, their grantee organizations and guided by the need for measurable results, something they felt had been lacking in prior HIV interventions. The use of performance-based financing, attached to a technical intervention like MSM testing, promised to allay these concerns; but, at the same time, they led to unsavory practices, such as "repeat testers" and other forms of deception by grantees, to gain additional performance incentives. In contrast, ACF initiated its MSM testing project as a response to discontented activists who desired community-oriented, peer-based testing options by and for MSM. For ACF, testing became envisioned and promoted as a source of empowerment and became part of a narrative that encouraged MSM to take control of their health by getting tested and knowing their status. This narrative stood in contrast to the prioritization of performance-based financing and performance targets underscored in the Health Fund's testing initiative. Despite these differences, both testing initiatives demonstrated the adaptability of HIV testing as a powerful technology that does and can do things beyond its intended purpose, as I explore in more detail in the next chapter.

MAKING UP
(AND MAKING AVAILABLE)
MSM IN CHINA

AFTER DINNER LATE ONE EVENING IN 2011, Zhang Li and I started talking about the push to scale up testing among MSM as we made our way to the subway station in Beijing. I recounted to her a meeting I attended earlier that day at the Health Fund to address some of the issues emerging from its HIV program. The main focus of the meeting was tackling the ongoing problem of "repeat testers" (see chapter 1) after a number of Health Fund grantees had been caught engaging in this practice so as to collect additional performance incentives. Zhang Li, who was consulting on the Health Fund's HIV program at the time, in addition to serving as a core member of the ACF team, did not seem surprised by this; she had come across similar incidents, she told me. As we discussed this challenge, I naively pointed out what I thought to be conflicting stakes generated by the performance incentives. The payment per test and per HIV-positive test structure clearly encouraged grantees to increase the number of HIV cases identified, even if this meant manufacturing the numbers to show false increases. But, I speculated, "If you wanted to control the epidemic, wouldn't you hope to find fewer cases (assuming the numbers were accurate)?" After all, I recalled, this intervention to expand MSM testing came out of anxiety around the increasing rates of HIV among the MSM population. It was implemented to bring down HIV prevalence.

In response, Zhang Li explained the public health logic behind the push to increase testing. The need to identify more cases, she clarified, is because "there is such limited knowledge about MSM in the country that the detection of more cases [among them] actually signals that the epidemic has been brought under control." Indeed, public health literature has long extolled the potential benefits of expanded testing and treatment approaches to controlling epidemics with an eye toward preventing secondary transmissions. In the case of HIV, this strategy can be especially helpful if targeted to groups like MSM, given their capacity to act as a "bisexual" bridge to the heterosexual population.[1] Zhang Li's reasoning reflected the public health script for Chinese MSM: that because they do not identify or acknowledge their same-sex attraction, and choose to remain in heterosexual lifestyles as is socially expected of them, they remain a "hidden" population that is neither visible nor identifiable to others. Their "invisibility" not only makes prevention difficult but further amplifies concerns that MSM's same-sex sexual practices may lead to a generalized epidemic that will ultimately be more difficult to contain.

Her argument was well taken, and I nodded in agreement. However, I pointed out that according to the most recent public health data I came across at the time, heterosexual contact was the leading route of trans-mission for HIV, not homosexual contact. I asked, in light of this data, isn't the anxiety around MSM misdirected? Zhang Li explained that "even though the numbers point to heterosexuals, they are really just men who don't admit to their *shenfen* [identity]," reiterating the public health script around their sexual behaviors. She noted that most of the men who came into the Chinese CDC for testing did not identify publicly as tongzhi or any other same-sex sexual identity but rather presented themselves as heterosexual, a complaint I often heard from CDC staff. Zhang Li described how "there is a genuine fear within the public health community that the epidemic will explode among MSM because we simply don't know how many more infected men are *out there* [empha-sis added]," again underscoring the urgency of scaling up MSM testing.

Zhang Li's attention to the possibility of more HIV-positive men "out there" was particularly striking to me, as if there might be a sur-plus of infected and infecting MSM bodies circulating among the gen-eral population. This notion called up, for me, an image of the "sur-feit" of poor and rural bodies once seen to be an obstacle to China's modernization and that necessitated and justified state interventions (Anagnost 1995; see also Greenhalgh and Winckler 2005). Just as the state stepped in to restrict the number of births allowable among rural farmers to meet national modernization goals, so global health donors intervened to expand MSM testing to control the HIV epidemic. In both instances, an imagery of excess galvanized massive endeavors by heightening senses of urgency around bodies, whether of peasants or of MSM. I started to consider the HIV testing intervention as an effort to identify MSM, to draw them out, and to make them visible to the state as MSM.

In this chapter, I examine how "making up MSM" became pivotal to the push to scale up testing among MSM in China. By making up, I refer to the process of instilling in these men a selfhood whereby they accept their sexual attraction to other men and their HIV risk as part and parcel of that desire. I show how this selfhood is cultivated through interactions of *ziworentong* (self-affirmation) intended to help men accept and even embrace their same-sex desires as a way to promote safe sexual choices, such as getting tested for HIV. The notion of *ziworentong* translates more directly to "self-identity" or "accepting one's identity." I suggest here that the process of fostering this selfhood entails much more than adopting an identity. Rather, the way *ziworentong* was incorporated into HIV testing projects insisted upon an acceptance and valorization of men's same-sex desires, which thereby not only reconfigured how they conceived of themselves but shaped how they acted as responsible citizens.

Here I draw on Ian Hacking's (1986; see also Sangaramoorthy and Benton 2012) notion of "making up people" to think through how counting practices such as those motivated by performance metrics create new categories of people, people who learn to have particular relations to themselves and ways to be. By linking performance-based financing to making up MSM, I demonstrate how enumeration practices have shaped the need to produce an "MSM" selfhood by which men are able to be mobilized to act and get tested voluntarily. Finding MSM, a key component to expanded HIV testing, was contingent upon having a population to count, and be counted, in performance metrics.

MSM IN HIDING AND THE PROBLEM OF TESTING MSM

Although scaling up MSM testing in China seemed like a promising strategy for meeting public health goals, they elicited a more pragmatic issue for donors, namely, the Health Fund and ACF. The problem was how to mobilize MSM to get tested voluntarily. Certainly, the imagery of infected/ing MSM bodies "out there" played a powerful role in motivating testing endeavors in the country by underscoring the "hiddenness" of the population. Yet, regardless of how motivated community-based organizations were in reaching out to MSM, there remained two key challenges to testing MSM in China. First is the flexibility by which men understand their sexuality. As I described in the introduction, many Chinese men maintain a "double life," performing a public heterosexual masculinity while engaging in same-sex sexual activities in private. This strategy allows these men to adhere to social expectations for Chinese men and pursue their same-sex desires simultaneously.

This sexual flexibility leads to a second issue: sexual identities and practices among MSM in China are diverse and not always concordant. Take, for example, Ah Zhen, whom I met in a meeting I attended in 2011 as part of an ACF monitoring trip to northeastern China. This small gathering had been organized by one of ACF's grantees, Lan Ai (hereinafter referred to as Blue Heart), a community-based organization providing sexual health services to MSM. In addition to participating in ACF's Test, Treat, and Prevent project, Blue Heart had at the time initiated a ziworentong project as a complement to its testing, something Jonah advocated to ACF's grantees. The meeting, at which Jonah, Zhang Li, and I were present, also included two staff from Blue Heart and three HIV-positive men who had been tested and diagnosed by Blue Heart as part of ACF's testing project, and who had joined the ziworentong initiative.

The three HIV-positive participants ranged in age and sexual orientation: two of the men were in their mid-twenties, and both identified as tongzhi. Ah Zhen, an older man in his mid-forties, acknowledged his same-sex sexual activities and considered himself a part of that community, though he never identified with any same-sex sexual identity and maintained a heterosexual lifestyle in accordance with the social norms he felt were expected of him. The two young men revealed that they had not yet fully disclosed their HIV statuses to their family members. One of the young men had shared his HIV status with his sister, but not his sexual preference, a common scenario I encountered. He explained that he still planned to get married one day and start a family. The other young man, having contracted HIV from his one and only sexual partner, had not told his parents, with whom he lived, either his sexuality or his HIV status.

In contrast, Ah Zhen shared with us that he had, in his words, been open about his HIV-positive status with everyone in his life: "Everyone knows: my friends, my past sexual partners, I'm out in the community, I don't hide it." He made it clear to us that he had already notified all of his past sexual partners of his HIV status, or *pengyou* (a euphemism for same-sex partners that translates into "friends"), and that he intended to do the same to all of his future sexual partners, indicating that he planned to continue his sexual activities with men.

Ah Zhen then shared a recent experience he had had with his son that gave him pause regarding transmissibility. "I was playing outside with my son," he recounted, "when I accidentally injured myself and began to bleed. I was terrified to touch my son because I didn't want to infect him since I was HIV-positive [*ganranzhe*]." At his retelling of this story, Jonah expressed confusion given Ah Zhen's statement that "everyone knows"; Ah Zhen admitted that he had not informed his spouse or his son of his HIV or sexual status, even as he insisted that he was out in the community, drawing a careful distinction between his public and personal lives. He assured us, nonetheless, that he was unlikely to transmit the virus to his wife since "we stopped having sex a long time ago." He added, "I thought about telling my wife, and I asked my best friend about it, but he told me not to do it. He thought it might be better not to say anything." Ah Zhen, like the others, had chosen not to share his HIV status with the individuals most present in his life.

Ah Zhen's story perfectly illustrates why making up MSM became so important to HIV testing in China. He represents a large number of MSM "in hiding," that is, men who strategically remain hidden but who can be made aware of their HIV risk as MSM and thus mobilized to get tested. At the time of our meeting, Ah Zhen carefully demarcated boundaries between the social spheres he inhabited, choosing to be "out" about his statuses (HIV and sexual) in what he considered to be his "community" of other men who engage in sex with men, and yet remaining silent about these statuses in his "public," heteronormative sphere. That Ah Zhen was able to traverse heterosexual and same-sex social worlds was not unique and was reminiscent of gay men in the early to mid-twentieth century described by George Chauncey (1994), men who perfected how to "pass" in New York City's then-straight spaces. Ah Zhen's "passing" was what rendered him, and many others in China like him, difficult to access. Whether because they were difficult to access, because they were understood to be "hidden," or both, Ah Zhen and the others triggered public health anxieties.

HIV TESTING AS COMING OUT

The ability to render MSM like Ah Zhen countable, and, relatedly, visible, speaks to the versatility of the HIV test as a technology that draws out "hidden" men, much as it does the HIV virus. Diagnostic tests developed in the 1980s gradually improved the accuracy of detecting HIV antibodies in the blood, thereby making the virus, and the person carrying the virus, known and knowable. Over the years, HIV tests underwent a series of improvements to enhance their capabilities, including the development of a rapid HIV test for responding to emergency situations (e.g., body fluid exposure, emergency room settings, clinic use; see Alexander 2016). The HIV test, to be clear, did not emerge to track and surveil populations per se but to make visible the presence of the virus in individual bodies.

And yet, this technology quickly showed itself to be productive beyond its epidemiological origins. Catherine Waldby (1996, 105) argued that the HIV test performed multiple duties as a "diagnostic technology for clinical medicine, a surveillance technology for epidemiology, and a disciplinary technology for the medico/social management of the infected." She noted that the HIV test acts as a "bio-administrative regime" that, once yielding a positive result, triggers a series of "confessional" tests for identity, drawing out a person's history in order to place the person into the appropriate public health category for risk transmission: sex workers, MSM, people who inject drugs. It is likely that this kind of surveillance further compelled Chinese MSM to present as heterosexuals and mask their same-sex sexual behaviors before public health authorities. As Waldby wrote, "the HIV test is the central technology in the biomedical mapping of the virus's presence in the body politic" (105). In this regard, the HIV test was and is a technology of the self (see Foucault 1988).

Consider, then, how HIV testing could be useful for drawing out MSM "in hiding," as became clear to me during a trip I took with ACF in May 2011. As a last-minute stop during one of ACF's regional monitoring trips to meet with grantees, Jonah, Zhang Li, and I decided to travel to a small, peripheral city in central China to meet with Li Qian, an administrator with the local Chinese CDC office. Li Qian, having heard about ACF's Test, Treat, and Prevent project from one of ACF's grantees in a nearby city, reached out to Jonah to discuss the possibility of starting the initiative in her city. Jonah initially expressed skepticism about starting a testing project in that particular city: "It's a strange place to do testing for MSM," he remarked. I admit that I shared his reservations given the demographic of the epidemic in that region. Li Qian resided in a place that had experienced an HIV outbreak in the 1990s resulting from commercial blood and plasma stations. This epidemic affected thousands of rural farmers, who contracted HIV as a consequence of unsanitary practices in the collection of blood and plasma (see Rosenthal 2000, 2001). The majority of HIV cases in the region remained concentrated among rural, heterosexual farmers. Nonetheless, in her correspondence with Jonah, Li Qian insisted that MSM testing was needed, thereby convincing Jonah, at the very least, to schedule a meeting.

In the meeting, Jonah conveyed his reservations about starting an MSM testing project in the city, asking, "Is there even a population to do rapid HIV testing here?" Li Qian replied that she counted "probably fifty or so" men in the area, speculating that "there are probably more, but they are just not out or visible." She admitted that she herself had only recently encountered this population; prior to that, she "had no idea that this group even existed." Li Qian had become a key resource for MSM in this area, providing the kind of care and support they needed in a place where an "MSM community" was not yet realized. As Li Qian interacted more and more with these men, she became sympathetic to their struggles, and she recognized the absence of community and local groups to support them. She suggested to Jonah, Zhang Li, and I that starting an MSM testing project may "actually help more of them come out and get tested."

I read Li Qian's motivation to join ACF's project as a sign of her caring for the men with whom she worked, along with her awareness that there may be more infected/ing MSM bodies "out there," just not "out or visible," as she had said. Indeed, by the end of our discussion, she estimated that "there may be about a hundred or more MSM in the area," suggesting that many of these men went to nearby cities to participate in same-sex sexual activities.

In building on Waldby's insights, I suggest that HIV tests not only mark bodies in the body politic; they also act as an instrument to draw out and standardize MSM, that is, to render them visible and countable in the same way they do HIV antibodies in the blood. To public health experts, men like Ah Zhen pose a challenge to prevention and control because they elide detection and enumeration. That is, they "pass." And yet, I argue that such men increasingly are made to count, if only because the performance-based practices adopted by global health donors (like the Health Fund) require new categories of people to count and new ways to count those people. Testing interventions work in concert with the MSM category to standardize and transform these men's lived differences into "interchangeable counts, data points, or goals" (Biruk 2019, 200).

Following our meeting, Jonah did not approve Li Qian's request for testing, although he remained sympathetic to her concerns. Instead, he suggested she initiate a ziworentong project for the men in her city. He suggested that this initiative might be more appropriate in light of the small number of MSM in the area, because "the point of ziworentong is to build rapport among the men to help them accept their same-sex desires, thereby helping them protect themselves against HIV." In other words, he seemed to say, self-affirmation is the first step toward getting men tested.

THE PROBLEM (AND PRESSURES) OF TESTING MSM

In the case of the Health Fund, testing initiatives came up against a series of challenges from the beginning (see chapter 1). In addition to the issue of "repeat testers" and other forms of subversive practice, another sort of problem started to emerge during my time in the field. In some of the Health Fund's more peripheral program sites, organizers were returning abysmally low testing and detection rates. In one city in southern China, the testing rates had been so low that program staff brought on an independent consultant to conduct a rapid assessment of the site and to recommend solutions that would boost its testing and detection rates.

That consultant, Ah Gu, spent nearly a week at the program site mapping out local public health infrastructures and social terrains that may be pertinent to MSM testing. As a self-identified tongzhi and the director of one of the largest nongovernmental organizations (NGOs) serving tongzhi in the country, and having participated in multiple HIV testing initiatives, including the Health Fund's, Ah Gu was uniquely qualified to carry out this assessment. In addition to meeting with relevant government players, such as the Chinese CDC and other public health agencies, Ah Gu interacted with local businesses and community-based organizations serving MSM to better understand the "culture" *(wenhua)* of MSM in this city, and he accompanied the Chinese CDC on its regular outings to conduct HIV outreach and testing among MSM.

Shortly after Ah Gu completed his evaluation, I traveled with Yang Xia (the Health Fund program officer introduced in chapter 1) and other staff from the Health Fund to the program site in June 2011. Having just barely made it onto one of the last flights out of Beijing that day, it was nearly 9:00 P.M. by the time we dropped off our belongings at a hotel and headed out to meet Ah Gu. Tired, we opted to stay close to the hotel, because we had an early start the next morning. We ended up at a dingy but cozy roadside stall offering fresh coconuts. Eager to know what Ah Gu found, Yang Xia dispensed with the pleasantries and immediately asked to hear his preliminary thoughts.

Ah Gu started out by telling us a story of an encounter he had had the night before our arrival. He had accompanied the local Chinese CDC on one of its monthly outings to carry out testing among MSM. The activity included setting up a small HIV testing station outside the entrance of the only gay bar in the city. There the CDC staff asked patrons to submit to an HIV test in lieu of the entrance fee.[2] Ah Gu had taken this opportunity to chat with some of the young men waiting in line to enter (and get tested) and asked if they knew why they were getting tested. One of the men said he knew they were getting an HIV and syphilis test, but he offered little more information beyond that. Ah Gu then followed up by asking the man how he might react if the test turned out to be positive. "He didn't say anything, he went blank," Ah Gu told us; "[the man] had never even thought about the possibility of testing positive."

Following this story, Ah Gu gave us his insights into why the program site returned such low testing and detection rates. "The problem is that there is no community [*shequ*] here, only a population [*renqun*]," he remarked. He elaborated by explaining how many of the men in the area lacked a clear understanding of why HIV testing is and should be an important endeavor for them as MSM. This "ignorance" could be attributed, partly, to the CDC's approach to administering testing,

which Ah Gu described as extending a technical act into a "key population" of men who shared no sociality and had no understanding of
their HIV risk as MSM. In this scenario, testing functioned as a clinical act, not as a preventative one that could be part and parcel of self-
care. Furthermore, Ah Gu clarified that with the on-site testing activities, much like the one at the bar, there is no counseling or individual
consultation carried out between the CDC staff conducting the testing
and the men getting tested. Therefore many men fail to understand the
linian (philosophy) behind the practice, and testing becomes, simply,
about taking blood. For this reason, Ah Gu noted, he often heard men
referring to testing as *caixue* (collecting blood) rather than *jiance* (testing for the purposes of prevention and care).

Yang Xia reiterated Ah Gu's assessment, lamenting that many of the
Health Fund's grantees seemed to care about little else than meeting
their performance targets in order to collect performance incentives,
hence the problem of "repeat testing." She acknowledged that in their
HIV program, the work of testing had become more about metrics than
about doing something meaningful for their communities. From her
perspective, the philosophy behind testing often got lost in the push for
numbers, and community-based organizations didn't always grasp why
the numbers mattered for more than the performance incentives. "It is
not about testing," she reiterated. "It is about knowing your HIV status,
early detection, and early treatment in order to reduce transmission."
To be sure, I often observed Health Fund staff display frustration at the
grantees' seeming lack of understanding around testing. I once heard a
program officer comment that community-based organizations seemed
to think that testing "is just to get money" and perceived the Health
Fund to be "just a bank."

Ah Gu expanded on Yang Xia's observations to further articulate
his point about the need for a community. In the absence of a community, MSM are unlikely to be mobilized for testing because they do
not feel connected to or belonging in a community of others "just like
them." Nor are they likely to understand the meaning behind getting
tested as MSM as a form of self-care. This principle is illustrated in
Robert Lorway and Shamshad Khan's (2014) study of Avahan, a Gates
Foundation–supported HIV program in India. Lorway and Khan described the distinctions that outreach workers made between men who
can be mobilized in HIV interventions as part of "the" community

(i.e., men who could be targeted for interventions) and those who cannot be mobilized because "they are non-community—they just fuck and go" (60). In China, as in India, MSM cannot be moved to action if they do not see themselves as belonging to a wider community in which testing is made meaningful, as an act of caring for the self and of caring for one's community. Community thereby functions not only as a space of shared affinity but as a technical site of mobilization (McKay 2018).

The issue facing the program site at which Ah Gu consulted was that many of the community-based organizations tasked with testing MSM were founded only after the Health Fund started its program there and emerged primarily for the purpose of testing MSM (I discuss this issue in more detail in chapter 4). Unlike Bright Love, with its new office space and movie room and a lounge filled with colored sofas for socializing and creating sociality (see the introduction), these organizations tested—only. Moreover, many of these newly formed organizations had been started with the help of the Chinese CDC and remained strongly affiliated with it. As Ah Gu explained,

> here is your challenge: volunteers [from grassroots groups] working with the Chinese CDC may say to men, "I'm tongzhi," but other men may perceive the volunteers as government staff and not as part of a *shequ* [community]. This is because these groups only exist inside the Health Fund's program, but they don't do anything outside of it. They were created specifically to implement HIV testing for international donors, but they have nothing else to fall back on once this money disappears. Instead, these groups should be thinking about helping MSM come out.

His commentary underlines a key point about MSM testing: that MSM, and MSM communities, must be made up—or, in Ah Gu's words, MSM must see themselves as MSM and as members of an MSM community— for HIV testing to succeed, or at least to see increased rates. After all, why would men go to a community-based organization targeting MSM if they do not see themselves as MSM, do not see themselves as at risk for HIV, and do not perceive the organizations' leaders and staff as representing the interests of a community of others like them?

The recommendation offered by Ah Gu at the end of his consultation encouraged the Health Fund to invest in a ziworentong project at the site, to develop an MSM selfhood so that men might recognize their HIV risk as part and parcel of their same-sex desires. He suggested that such an initiative could "help [the men] protect themselves a little more, because they might have more confidence and self-assurance" with which to make safe sexual choices. Ah Gu intentionally and strategically linked self-knowledge to self-care, and ultimately to HIV testing. Ziworentong is not just about self-affirmation. It is a technique for reconfiguring social relations to produce a new community. It is noteworthy to recall that Ah Gu's recommendations were made for another purpose: to increase testing and detection rates among MSM for the Health Fund's HIV program.

* * * * *

The Health Fund's concerns with increasing testing and detection rates at its program sites put additional pressure on community-based organizations to step up their testing efforts. It was, after all, to these groups that the Health Fund and other donors (including ACF) turned to carry out the actual promotion and delivery of testing. Throughout the course of my fieldwork, I consistently encountered complaints from community-based organizations related to meeting performance targets for the Health Fund's program. For many, meeting or exceeding these targets determined the likelihood of obtaining future grants (see also Miller 2016).

The prevailing sentiments among many leaders and staff of community-based organizations are aptly conveyed in the frustration-filled criticism I once heard the director of an NGO direct at the Health Fund: "Stop demanding quotas and other kinds of indicators that place burdens on us but don't actually help the community." But as Jonah often reminded ACF's grantees, there are different stakes involved for different players in the fight against HIV. "The goal of the Health Fund's program," Jonah reminded, "is to reduce transmission, not to do guanhuai [care]." He proceeded to admonish community-based organizations for "always complaining that you want donors to give you money, but it is not always about your needs and what you want to do." Instead, Jonah argued the donors also have their needs and their challenges, such as doing evaluations for which metrics are needed; otherwise, "how will they know if their programs are effective?" He reminded his audience that "a donor isn't just going to give you money because you want it and trust you will get things done," perhaps gesturing to ACF's own collection of numbers in its testing project.

For some community-based organizations, the need for metrics translated into more pressure to meet performance targets. A staff member at Bright Love once described to me, "Our group is required to conduct five hundred to six hundred tests per project period; we are constantly under pressure to increase the number of tests we do for the Health Fund." And yet, for others, there was a more meaningful reason to scale up testing among MSM: to save lives. For many of the leaders and staff of organizations with whom I met, the push to get men tested formed a key part of self-care, extending beyond performance targets and other forms of incentivization.

MSM AS BIOSEXUAL CITIZENS

The challenges of HIV testing among Chinese MSM often led me to ask, How do MSM come to understand themselves to be at risk for HIV? How can men be motivated to get tested voluntarily on the basis of that risk? In the social sciences, anthropologists have long been interested in citizenship projects organized around biological forms of existence. These ideas are clearly articulated in Nikolas Rose and Carlos Novas's (2005) use of biological citizenship to describe projects that reshape how individuals are thought about and acted upon as citizens, converging around their biological existence.[3] Biological citizenship projects are not necessarily imposed from above; rather, they can be "individualizing and collectivizing" (441) insofar as the enterprising self becomes the subject of self-care and self-management and must act responsibly as part of greater collectivities formed around a biologically shared identity. This is what Paul Rabinow (1996) calls biosociality.

These kinds of projects, argue Rose and Novas, are administered through multiple channels. In addition to the more traditionally authoritative platforms, such as medical reports or health education, an increasing number of people are seeking out information from media outlets like the internet. Priscilla Song (2017) examined how "biomedical self-shaping" (Rose and Novas 2005, 446) was mediated through online communities like CareCure, a discussion forum dedicated to spinal cord injuries. She illustrated how the forum had come to play a powerful role in producing alternative forms of "patient-driven knowledge production" (26) by publishing personal narratives written by its members. These narratives, and the knowledge readers and writers alike derived from them, generated new forms of identity, sociality, and activism among individuals who saw other forum participants as "just like them." Individuals on this platform often used "biologically colored languages" (Rose and Novas 2005, 445) to describe and understand parts of their identities.

Social encounters, both online and offline, work to actively reshape how persons come to understand themselves as biological beings and to act upon themselves in biological ways. Joseph Dumit (2012) described such self-shaping in his study of pharmaceutical companies. He demonstrated how direct-to-consumer advertisements compelled nonsick consumers to intervene upon their potentially sick bodies as if their bodies were concealing disease from them. Dumit argued that the goal of these advertisements was to convert knowing into doing. Thus the advertising campaigns first produced a biomedical subjectivity through which nonpatients began to identify as patients, and second, the campaigns relocated responsibility for managing one's health from the medical professional to the individual. By the end, individuals were empowered to take control of their health by demanding their right to pharmaceuticals.

More recently, some scholars have turned to the notion of biosexual citizenship (Norton quoted in Epstein 2018) to describe citizenship projects that are organized around sexuality.[4] Steven Epstein (2018) used this concept to illustrate how pleasures and risks associated with sexuality are applied in public health and by public health authorities to define sexual rights and responsibilities. He traced the genealogies of social hygiene and sexual health to show how sexual citizenship became central to conceptions of being a good citizen. His ideas have been elaborated upon by other scholars who have shown, for example, how public health strategies like preexposure prophylaxis (PrEP) or treatment as prevention produce biosexual citizens who define their sexual rights and responsibilities through the risks associated with their particular sexualities. MSM, for example, who do not adhere to the strict regimes of PrEP were seen by others in their communities to violate the terms of this citizenship and risked being positioned as "standing against health" (Orne and Gall 2019, 644).

The concept of biosexual citizenship is useful for understanding how forms of biological and sexual self-shaping compelled men like

Xiao Lin, a self-identified tongzhi I met in October 2011, to get tested for HIV for the first time. Xiao Lin learned he was HIV-positive in 2008, and by the time I met him, he had separated from the *bf* (boyfriend) from whom he contracted HIV. He explained that the idea that he might be at risk for or even contract HIV had never entered into his mind. It was only after he encountered HIV testing campaigns promoted by community-based organizations targeting MSM that he chose to be tested. He shared that "up until 2006 or 2007, no one knew anything about *aizibing* [AIDS], especially in our *quanzi* [circle]."[5] He admitted that he "always thought about it as something far away [*li women hen yuan*], that it could never happen to us." Instead, he felt a kind of social and spatial distance from the epidemic, as if contracting HIV was something that "only happened in big cities like Beijing or Shanghai, not in smaller places where we are."

Only in the past few years had information about HIV begun circulating in Xiao Lin's community. "Prior to that," he noted, "no one knew anything about condoms or prevention. But nowadays, everyone knows." His supposition that HIV was something far away was a notion I encountered often among the MSM I met. During the time I spent in a clinic where MSM sought treatment for conditions associated with anal sex, many of the men with whom I spoke expressed surprise at having contracted HIV. Many admitted, like Xiao Lin, that they viewed HIV as "something far away from us." Other authors of public health studies, likewise, have documented the low perception of risk among MSM, identifying this as a key factor in low testing rates among MSM (Choi et al. 2006; Huang et al. 2012; Tao et al. 2014; Wei et al. 2014). The director of a community-based organization with which I worked attributed many MSM's imagined distance from HIV as a reason for the high number of men getting tested and testing positive for the first time. "They just never thought to be tested before," the director explained.

Getting tested for the first time almost always required men to recognize themselves as MSM and as at risk for HIV, much as Xiao Lin did. The shift in understanding of one's self, and of one's inclusion in the MSM category, was crucial for HIV testing initiatives, as it made men newly available and amenable to such testing. In China, what facilitated these reconceptualizations of self were the ziworentong initiatives that aimed to instill in men an acceptance of their same-sex

desires along with the understanding that their same-sex sexual practices placed them at risk for HIV. By examining how these initiatives
played out, I demonstrate the kinds of work that went into making up
MSM and making men available to the HIV testing markets that proliferated under performance-based financing regimes. I suggest that as
more and more MSM voluntarily sought out testing, they were readily transformed into commodities of care, commodities that fueled the
HIV testing markets.

ACF AND ZIWORENTONG

Shortly after I arrived in China in fall 2010, I was given the opportunity
to attend one of ACF's ziworentong training workshops. These events
were held regularly throughout the year to guide staff and volunteers
from community-based organizations to initiate the ziworentong project in their own communities. The workshop was a form of "training of
trainers" that was by then a mainstay in health and development programs around the world. ACF provided small stipends to their grantees
to support local activities (e.g., testing, projects such as ziworentong),
in addition to funding grantee participation in these sponsored events.
Luckily, I had no plans that weekend, so when Jonah called to invite
me to participate in their two-day activity, I happily accepted. And so
it came to be that on a cold night in November, I found myself sitting
among a group of twenty or so men in a sparsely decorated, and somewhat damp, hotel conference room on the outskirts of Beijing. It had
been snowing that evening, and each of the men stomped his feet vigor-
ously as he entered to remove the ice from his boots. I sat to the side,
patiently, and yet anxiously, waiting for Jonah to begin. Finally, as the
last of the participants trickled in from the snow, Jonah stood up and
started the workshop.

Without much fanfare, Jonah gave a quick introduction to ACF and
the ziworentong project, providing few details about the goals of the
initiative, before launching into the first activity. He split the participants into three smaller groups of men and designated a preassigned
facilitator for each group before sending two of the three groups off into
nearby rooms. For no other reason than convenience, I opted to stay
with the group that remained in the room where I sat already. Before
starting the small-group activity, Jonah asked us to place the chairs in
a circle so that we all faced each other. Doing so, he clarified, fostered

intimacy and belonging, helping everyone to feel included as part of the community that this project aimed to generate.

Once the chairs were properly arranged and everyone was seated, Jonah paused for a moment, then asked, "What was your best and worst sexual experience?"

Silence and awkwardness filled the air. No one responded. A few of the participants, myself included, traded puzzled glances, unsure of what to say. Following what seemed like several minutes of quiet, one man softly said, "The worst sexual experience I had was with a man I met on QQ (an instant messaging service)."[6] Taking a deep breath, he continued: "I had been chatting with this man online for a few weeks, and we decided to meet in person. I took a train to another city where we had arranged to meet in a hotel. When he got there, I told this man that I didn't want to have sex immediately. Instead, he gave me a hand job [da feiji] a couple of times, and then we went to sleep. I felt bad about the entire thing because it seemed like he was only interested in having sex and that was it."[7]

This man's story seemed to be the opening salvo needed for the other participants to share. One by one, the other men began revealing their own stories of intimacy, some tender, some not so tender, though all expressed feelings of pleasure and pain produced in those sexual encounters. The "worst sexual experiences" the men described sometimes brought into sharp relief the best sexual experiences, ones that mostly evoked moments of caring—for others and for themselves. An older man in his mid-fifties shared that he "came into this circle" (zou jin zhege quanzi) after being coerced into sexual relations with his employer when he was a teenager. The director of the company for which he worked at the time got him drunk one night and forced him to engage in sexual intercourse. He and the director ended up in a relationship for the next three years, although the man admitted that the director often threatened him, forbidding him to leave or to tell anyone about the relationship. This man, who identified neither as tongzhi nor by any other sexual identity, joked halfheartedly that this was how he bai wan, or "turned gay," suggesting that he had sex with men as a result of this violent sexual encounter.[8] He confessed that his feelings for his former partner remain unresolved: "In looking back on it, I loved him and I hated him for what he did to me. But there were good times, too, when he was really loving toward me."

Another participant, a soft-spoken young man in his mid-twenties, described his turbulent three-year relationship with the partner from whom he contracted HIV. At times the partner was violent, and in other moments he was so tender that, the young man explained, he could not bring himself to leave; therefore he stayed with this man despite the partner's possessiveness. "This isn't just a bad relationship," Jonah remarked. "It is a bad life [shenghuo]," indicating how this decision impacted the rest of this man's life in permanent, not temporary, ways. His remark underlined the aim of ziworentong; to alter how men valued their lives, as men who desire other men, and recognized their HIV risk as part of that desire. This point is particularly salient given that many of the participants that night shared that they contracted HIV as a consequence of the sexual encounters they described in the meeting. Yet another man spoke of a past relationship that had its tumultuous moments since his partner was "out" and he himself was not at the time. Despite this, the man recounted a favorite moment that did not involve sex at all but rather two weeks of sharing a bed and developing an intimacy before initiating a sexual relationship.

After each of the participants in our small group (myself excluded; see chapter 5 for my explanation) shared his story, Jonah asked the participants, "What do all these stories have to do with HIV prevention?" Just as in the beginning, his question was met with silence. No one, myself included, knew how to respond. Jonah then answered his question for us: "HIV prevention is not only about testing and safe sex; it is also about accepting ourselves."

* * * * *

The ziworentong project implemented by ACF started prior to the Test, Treat, and Prevent project as a way to assist MSM to work through and ideally come to embrace their same-sex desires. The project specifically targeted men considered to be part of the "hidden population" (yinxing renqun), requiring that at least 60 percent of ziworentong project participants come from this demographic. These were men who were less likely to frequent same-sex public spaces, such as bars, bathhouses, or parks. According to ACF, they were men who "may have difficulty accepting themselves [or] understanding their same-sex desires" and, as a result, may experience feelings of guilt or, in more serious cases, may abandon or give up on themselves. Many of the men participating in the ziworentong project remained in heterosexual relationships. These men, explained Jonah, were less likely to engage in safe sexual practices to "protect oneself" *(ziwo baohu)*.

After the project's initial three-year cycle, Jonah felt strongly enough about the positive benefits of the initiative to start promoting its implementation in conjunction with the Test, Treat, and Prevent project. Thus, by the time I was in the field, Jonah was regularly integrating ziworentong into the Test, Treat, and Prevent workshops, training grantees to initiate ziworentong in their communities at the same time that grantees were learning to implement testing technologies. The pairing of these two initiatives created a two-pronged approach to expanding MSM testing that, at the same time, reinforced ACF's core mission to empower individuals and communities to care for themselves.

The goals of the ziworentong project were threefold: to increase participants' self-confidence, to expand their social networks and support systems, and to improve their awareness of HIV and other sexual risks. These aims reflect a series of assumptions that guided the project from its inception: (1) that men do not accept their same-sex attraction and, as a result, (2) that men are not aware of their HIV risks; as such, (3) men may engage in risky sexual practices. Ziworentong therefore was meant to help MSM develop a positive and healthy understanding of themselves as same-sex-desiring men by helping them cultivate a social network of others "just like them" in the hope that a positive attitude and stronger social ties would aid them in making safe sexual decisions.

The creation of safe spaces for men to share their personal stories, much like the one I described earlier, was central to the ziworentong project. Jonah hoped that in these spaces, men would learn to identify the sexual practices that make them vulnerable to HIV, both emotionally and otherwise. They would learn, at least in ACF's iteration, through heart-to-heart talks *(tanxin)*. *Tanxin* was popularized in China as a form of talk therapy counseling that could validate a person's experience and lead to healing by allowing an individual to express their innermost thoughts to a counselor or therapist (Yang 2015). This process worked to enable individuals to take responsibility for and seek out solutions to their problems (Yang 2015). Jonah and others hoped that heart-to-heart talks, as a form of storytelling, would generate new selfhoods among MSM while helping men accept, and take responsibility for, their same-sex desires and sexual behaviors, and recognize their HIV risks. Unlike popular *tanxin* practices, however, rather than meeting individually or in groups with a counselor, the ziworentong project encouraged men to share their stories with their peers—that is, with other MSM.

The format of ziworentong was not unlike other "speaking-out" or "coming-out" activities mobilized by international organizations and which impelled forms of testimony. The Greater Involvement of People Living with HIV (GIPA) promoted by UNAIDS, for example, popularized the practice of sharing one's HIV-positive status publicly to empower people living with HIV and to combat stigma. Anthropologist Vinh-Kim Nguyen (2010) demonstrated in his research that speaking-out performances have been productive for consolidating a sense of self and identity among people living with HIV, which, in turn, gives these individuals greater access to international resources and other material benefits. Those who speak out, argued Adia Benton (2015), provide a template for how one should behave, articulating a set of expectations for becoming a responsible sexual citizen. "In disclosing," she wrote, "the HIV-positive individual responsibilizes—generates responsible acts—in both others and herself" (67). Disclosure also acts as a form of storytelling that, as Jie Yang (2015) suggested, reaffirms the individual while organizing new kinds of therapeutic governance that redirect accountability onto the individual but ignore the structural factors that contribute to things like unemployment—or, in the case of MSM, to contracting HIV.

To foster intimacy and trust among participants, ACF limited ziworentong cohorts to ten participants or fewer at any one time. In total, cohorts met four times—once per week—for four weeks in a row (additional weeks could be added, if needed). Each weekly session lasted for two hours, consisting of fifteen minutes for introductions, ninety minutes to discuss preassigned topics, and fifteen minutes for summaries and conclusions. The topics followed a particular sequence: week 1 opened with a discussion of participants' first sexual encounters (same-sex or not) as a way to reflect upon the effects of sex on their lives. In week 2, participants explored the "inner me and outer me," meaning their public and private personas, which could at times contradict each other, while also reflecting different aspects of the self. This topic was included to help individuals reconcile the social pressures placed on them to act in ways that conflicted with their personal desires as MSM. Next, in week 3, participants shared their best and worst sexual experiences, as in the example I used earlier, to identify the positive and negative aspects of their sexual relations. The goal of this session was to help individuals develop a healthy and positive attitude toward sex that, ideally, would help them make safe sexual choices. Finally, in week 4, participants were asked to imagine their present and future lives, both as a reflection upon the past few weeks and to envision, as a group, what an ideal life could look like.

The sequence of topics was meant to facilitate an exploration of a range of issues that related to sex and that potentially encumbered MSM, ultimately affecting their sexual health choices. The goal of these sessions, Jonah explained, was to valorize same-sex desires through intimate discussions of participants' innermost sexual thoughts and experiences, but also to validate participants' fears and anxieties, with a community of peers present to support them. The ziworentong project was structured to ensure that the same group of men attended each weekly session for the entire project period, not only to foster a sense of community, but as a result of this solidarity, to compel men into action—to get tested for HIV as an act of self-care, for example. The aim of this project, Jonah asserted, was to "build a strong sense of self in all men who have sex with men in order to encourage safe sexual practices." By knowing how to protect ourselves, he assured his audiences, we do not need to be afraid of HIV.

"I AM A CARRIER . . ."

The notion of personal or individual responsibility was a key theme across many of ACF's projects, and this focus was adopted by a number of ACF's grantees as well. It was in yet another workshop in May 2011, just days after my meeting with Jonah, Zhang Li, and Li Qian described earlier, that I came to understand how HIV testing of MSM transitioned from a clinical intervention traditionally carried out in hospitals, clinics, and other laboratory settings into an act of personal empowerment and a reflection of emerging MSM selfhoods.

Up until the time of this particular workshop, my fieldwork had consisted primarily of nonclinical-based activities, including participating in workshops, conferences, and meetings and traveling with the Health Fund and ACF, in addition to the performance of routine office work. These activities proved exceedingly valuable to my learning about how the different pieces of HIV testing came together, but they also meant that I spent very little time in clinical settings, where HIV testing is typically administered. Over the course of my research, I came to realize that where testing took place mattered as much as the conditions under which it was administered. Testing, as I came to learn, was no longer limited to clinical contexts; rather, it had extended into social spaces, such as bars and bathhouses, where MSM congregated. In these encounters, where the clinical meets the social, testing came to take on a deeper meaning: as an act of self-care and self-knowledge and as an experience that bound HIV to MSM in inextricable ways.

Anthropologists have demonstrated that the workshop is a mobile technology that travels as a standard form of knowledge across diverse contexts (Nguyen 2010; see also Benton 2015; Biruk 2018; McKay 2018), not unlike the HIV test. The workshop is a space where social relations are reconfigured, consensus is manufactured, and individual and collective subjectivities are produced. For this reason, these types of gatherings have played an important role in making up MSM, as described with regard to ACF's ziworentong initiative.

The workshop I attended that spring was held in a hotel conference room in the city, a relatively common site for such events in China. Arriving early, Jonah, Zhang Li, and I settled into chairs at the side of the room, leaving the main floor for the MSM participants. The men trickled in one by one, and the room quickly filled with smoke, despite the "no smoking" sign prominently featured on the wall. Facilitating the workshop that night was Lao Ye, the director of an organization that was an ACF grantee. An older man, he identified as a tongzhi in certain spaces, although he remained married with children. Nevertheless, he played an active role in the local tongzhi community and considered himself part of that community. He introduced us to the Chinese CDC staff members who had just walked in and were settling next to us. I was initially unsure about why CDC staff might be attending the workshop, but the reason became clear once Lao Ye started the workshop. He announced to the audience that the CDC doctor would be providing HIV testing after the event to anyone interested.

The night started off with a discussion about STIs. For this activity, Lao Ye split participants into smaller breakout groups and asked each group to share among themselves what they knew about different infections. After ten minutes in the breakout sessions, the participants re-convened in the larger group and recounted their discussions. The aim of this exercise, explained Lao Ye, was to clear up any misconceptions the men may have about STIs. He acknowledged that many people have stereotypes about what it means to have AIDS, and he presented a series of photos that showed the more serious medical effects of the condition, not unlike what one might expect to see in a sex education class. He tried to ameliorate the impact of these photos by praising the medical and technological advancements of the past few decades, which meant that being HIV-positive is no longer a death sentence. Instead, he emphasized, it is important that men know how to check for symptoms. Lao Ye then described the different ways that HIV can, and cannot, be transmitted. Taken at face value, the exercise was unremarkable, and yet, it segued pointedly into the next activity: a conversation about sexual pleasure.

Lao Ye initiated this discussion by asking the men, "What parts of your body do you find most erotic and pleasurable?" His question was met with a mix of awkward silence and nervous giggling. Perhaps sensing the participants' apprehension, he explained the rationale behind this question: "The reason for this exercise is [for participants] to become comfortable with having erogenous zones and taking pleasure in your sexuality. It is about affirming your desires, and taking responsibility for yourself by using condoms and preventing HIV so you can continue to experience these pleasures."

He then repeated, in revised form, his question: "So, what are some of the most pleasurable ways you enjoy having sex?" After a few more seconds of silence, an older participant, a man in his fifties, offered an answer: "*mo doufu,*" he said, a term that literally translates to "making tofu" and refers to rubbing penises together. At his response, a few more participants joined in: "*da feiji,*" one man shouted, or "beating the plane," referring to manual stimulation of the penis. "Good!" Lao Ye encouraged, as the discussion became increasingly animated once the participants became more comfortable.

After the discussion of men's erotic zones, Lao Ye linked the transmission and prevention of HIV and STIs to pursuits of sexual pleasure. He asked participants to share why some men chose not to use condoms when having sex, hoping to elicit a deeper understanding among the men of the practices that put them at risk. One participant offered,

"You trust your partner, so you don't feel like you need a condom"; another stated, "Your partner doesn't want you to wear one." The reasons given by these men echoed Zheng Tiantian's ethnographic findings in her 2015 study of tongzhi. She argued that many men view condoms as a marker of infidelity; not using condoms reflected their love and mutual trust for each other, whereas the use of condoms indicated that the user is sexually active, promiscuous, and possibly diseased.

The exercises Lao Ye led were designed to encourage participants to understand sexual pleasure and sexual risk not as incompatible but rather as complementary. By linking men's erotic zones to steps taken to prevent and minimize HIV and STI transmission, the workshop had been designed to convince participants that to minimize risk is to pursue one's pleasure in a safe and responsible manner. The workshop guided men to recognize that as men who enjoy sex with other men, they must take steps to care for themselves, and to do this, they must first acknowledge their same-sex sexual pleasures. By linking men's sexual pleasures with sexual responsibility, and yoking the acts that men find enjoyable to information about why they are at risk when engaging in those activities unsafely, Lao Ye was prodding participants to act as responsible sexual citizens. This became especially apparent at the end of the workshop.

As if to bolster the process of "subjectification" (Dreyfus and Rabinow 1982) whereby men come into being as (bio)sexual citizens at risk for HIV and act responsibly in this capacity, Lao Ye concluded with a series of "I" statements that he reminded the men to say to themselves if they were, in fact, HIV-positive:

I am a carrier.
I have a high viral count.
I am more likely to have sores.

Lao Ye then invited the CDC doctor to set up a small HIV testing station at the conference table in the middle of the room. The doctor carefully prepped the table—lining up the test tubes, disposable needles, gauze, and other implements—while Lao Ye reminded men of the importance of getting tested and knowing one's status and handed out standardized questionnaires to gather information about the men's sexual histories. Slowly, the men started to line up to get tested. The first volunteer, a young man in his mid-twenties, stood up hesitantly and rolled up his sleeves before sitting down at the conference table with his arm extended. He turned away as the doctor prepped the needle, and then confessed, "I'm afraid of needles," just as the syringe punctured his arm and the blood quickly spilled into the tube. As I watched the vials grow in number, I realized how powerful HIV testing had become as a technology for drawing out, making up, and enumerating MSM.

Shortly after the testing began, I walked over to the organizer of the workshop, an ACF grantee, to ask about the event. He explained that the local Chinese CDC requested that they put together this workshop to recruit MSM to get tested, as part of the CDC's sentinel surveillance activities. He affirmed that the expenses associated with the workshop were paid by the Chinese CDC, while the labor to bring these men together was provided by their organization. He noted that this kind of arrangement, whereby the CDC contracts their group to coordinate activities and recruit MSM for testing, is not unusual. Indeed, I met many leaders of community-based organizations who participated in similar arrangements. And yet, I wondered whether these HIV tests would be counted by the organization toward meeting performance metrics and collecting performance incentives.

CONCLUSION

This chapter has examined how and why making up MSM has been pivotal to the success of scaling up MSM testing in China. The success of this intervention relied, in many ways, on having and locating a population of MSM to test. A key challenge for public health authorities, and that emerged for donors like the Health Fund while implementing MSM testing, had been how to access these men given their ability to remain "in hiding," as I describe in this chapter, that is, men who traverse heterosexual and same-sex social worlds. Many men do not perceive themselves to be at risk for HIV and are not always aware of the importance of getting tested as part of caring for the self. For this reason, ACF and, to some degree, the Health Fund, turned to practices of ziworentong, or self-affirmation, as a way to instill in these men an acceptance of their same-sex desires and a recognition of their HIV risk as part and parcel of their desires. The ziworentong initiative has been carried out primarily through workshops that served as a crucial space for generating new selfhoods and socialities among MSM, while also acting as a site for making up responsible (bio)sexual citizens among

MSM. As I have argued in this chapter, the making up of MSM has emerged partly out of the need to count MSM in testing initiatives like those of the Health Fund and ACF. And yet, as I discuss in the next chapter, this process has also transformed MSM into commodities of care by linking their bodies to performance incentives.

THREE

MARKETS OF AND
MARKETING TO MSM

"HOW DO WE MARKET our products [*chanpin*] to people? How do we demonstrate the quality of our services to the community? And how do we get the Chinese CDC to purchase our services?" These were just a few of the questions that Xiao Fu, the director of a community-based organization serving MSM in south central China, presented to a small gathering of staff and volunteers from MSM groups one night in 2011. This informal event had been organized by Jonah, the director of ACF, as part of a three-day workshop for ACF's Test, Treat, and Prevent project held quarterly for their grantees. I was there at the invitation of Jonah. After a long day of discussions and debates at the workshop, Jonah invited participants who wished to brainstorm ideas for promoting HIV testing in their communities to join an informal gathering to share and exchange their experiences. About fifteen of us came together and made our way to the main conference room, casually taking up seats wherever they were scattered.

Xiao Fu, an energetic young man apparently unfazed by the post-dinner lethargy affecting many of the rest of us, stood up and offered to start the dialogue. Peering out from behind his black-rimmed glasses, he asked participants for advice on how best to meet two goals he had for his organization: first, to expand its "client" base, as he termed it, referring to MSM seeking HIV testing services, and second, to attract the Chinese CDC to *goumai fuwu,* or "purchase," its testing services, a practice more formally described as social service contracting.[1]

Xiao Fu's use of "client" to describe men seeking HIV services drew my immediate attention. This discursive decision seemed to displace the men his organization served from the realms of public health (as patients) and development endeavors (as beneficiaries) to instead recast them as consumers in a market economy (Whyte et al. 2013). Indeed, that Xiao Fu chose the term *client,* not unlike many organizational leaders I encountered in the field, signaled to me a pivotal shift in the public health landscape of the country: that MSM groups were, increasingly, purveyors, in addition to providers, of HIV care. Xiao Fu, like many others leading similar groups, hoped to expand his organization's HIV testing services for MSM as a way of sustaining the organization's operations. Yet, he struggled to find effective ways to do this, and specifically to convince the Chinese CDC to contract services from his organization rather than from other groups.

One strategy Xiao Fu considered was to carry out "market research," or *shichang diaocha,* to generate data regarding the quality of his organization's services, which included rapid HIV testing as part of ACF's project. He suggested that this research could involve preparing questionnaires or surveys to give to men, or clients, to again use his term, who came into the organization for HIV testing, not unlike a kind of customer satisfaction form. Xiao Fu felt that "if we want people to believe in our work, and if we want to convince the Chinese CDC to purchase our services, then we need to provide some sort of evidence to demonstrate the value of our work." In other words, he and his team needed to produce numbers, and "good" numbers, that could do the work of marketing for them. Such numbers were especially important, he reminded us, because "we are not just selling our products to the government, we are selling them to the community [of MSM]." Numbers are performative; they do things, such as validate the quality of an organization's services, as in Xiao Fu's case. His motives for undertaking market research, and thereby generating "good" numbers, were dual: to show potential funders that investing in the organization is "worth it" and to instill trust among potential clients.

As I listened to the conversation that took place that night, I was struck by two thoughts. On one hand, I was genuinely impressed, if not somewhat confounded, by Xiao Fu's use of business jargon. His deft delivery of this parlance sounded more apropos to a corporate seminar and seemed, at times, anathema to a grassroots gathering. Of course, my surprise reflected my own naïveté with regard to how powerfully global health ideas have shaped local community landscapes and how quickly and seamlessly these discourses have made their way into everyday usage. Xiao Fu's adoption of business rhetoric was perfectly appropriate, if not inevitable, given the prominence of performance metrics that underpinned technocratic interventions like testing as prevention in China, as well as in global health writ large. On the other hand, I couldn't help but wonder how testing became both a health intervention meant to save lives and an economic enterprise promising financial gains. To be sure, the commitment to doing both—saving lives and earning profits—undergirds the philanthrocapitalist regime to which many global health donors ascribe (see chapter 1), and yet I was confused by the ease with which these dual commitments could coexist.

It is to the assimilation of business-, metrics-, and profit-driven practices across public health landscapes in China that I turn in this chapter. Here, I am especially interested in examining how scaling up HIV testing among MSM has altered the scope of prevention and other forms of HIV work possible in local public health spaces. That there has been such a narrowing of possibilities for HIV prevention work outside of testing in China helps to think about how technical interventions can shape individual and collective health practices in general. The rise of global health donors and their demand for metrics, argued Katerini Storeng and Dominique Béhague (2017), has profoundly limited the kinds of arguments and forms of evidence that count as authoritative in contemporary health debates. I show that these limitations have resulted from the scaling up of testing.

In what follows, I trace the implementation of social service contracting enacted by the Chinese CDC to scale up testing among MSM as a key public health strategy. By attending to these practices, I demonstrate how standardized interventions like MSM testing unfold within and in conjunction with local public health systems in China in ways that curtailed the kinds of interventions available to MSM and, in so doing, reconfigured what counts as HIV care. The social service contracts described in this chapter involve similar performance-based financing structures promoted by global health donors like the Health Fund; that they do underscores the capacity of business discourse to shape local health strategies. And while the majority of HIV financing in China now comes from the Chinese government and not international donors, as it once did, the shift to government-funded HIV service provisioning seems to dovetail well with the market reforms that have decentralized health care systems in the country.

SOCIAL SERVICE CONTRACTING IN CONTEXT

The pervasiveness of performance-based financing, utilized to scale up testing among MSM, did not arise from nowhere; rather, these schemes aligned to economic shifts already under way in China. Beginning with the postsocialist reforms in the late 1970s, Chinese officials have increased marketization, downsizing direct government intervention as part of a broader "small state, big society" vision (Irish, Salamon, and Simon 2009; Simon 2013; Teets 2012; Jia and Su 2009). This transition did not entail a withdrawal or attenuation of state powers but was marked instead by a shift from direct to indirect forms of governance, a devolution of responsibilities from central to local agencies, and the promotion of personal responsibility (Greenhalgh 2010). Reforms resulted in the privatization of many state-owned enterprises that once guaranteed the kinds of welfare benefits that inspired the Chinese idiom "eating from the iron rice bowl" *(tiefanwan)*. Gradually, the responsibility for delivering social services to the citizenry was relocated from the central government to already-constrained local governments with limited budgets.

Social service contracting emerged in the 1990s as a way for the central government to reduce the administrative workload in a cost-effective manner while also meeting citizens' needs. In effect, the government purchases social services (e.g., home care, elder care, legal aid, mental health services) from local social organizations; it is a system already well established in other countries. Arguably, social service contracting allows the Chinese government to adhere to its goals of bettering society while maintaining its political legitimacy for doing so (Liao, Zeng, and Zhang 2015; Jing 2008).[2]

Since the 1990s, social service contracting has evolved. Early phases loosely relied on arrangements of *guanxi*, or networks of personal relationships that operate as contemporary forms of patron-clientelism (Uretsky 2016). These interactions were undergirded not only by systems of reciprocity but also by relations of affect, affinity, and loyalty (Osburg 2013). The cultural embeddedness of *guanxi* meant that contracts were typically awarded to institutions with strong affiliations or ties to the government, even though these were often beset by poor performance, corruption, and little if any citizen participation (Jing and Chen 2012). As I discovered, such relationships continued to guide the administration of social service contracts in the HIV sector at the time of my fieldwork. Following the relative ineffectiveness of these arrangements, however, the Chinese government began attending to social service contracting in earnest, releasing a series of guidelines to formalize its implementation across all levels of government.

Key regulatory policies, such as the 1999 Competitive Bidding Law and the 2002 Government Procurement Law, were enacted, establishing rules for competitive bidding to improve fiscal transparency, accountability, and performance (Jing and Chen 2012). Additionally, the Guidance on Purchasing Services from Society explicitly identified social organizations (including nongovernmental, community-based, and grassroots) as one of the entities from which the government could contract. This policy marked an important step in the government's growing awareness that social organizations could play a pivotal role in delivering services, thereby filling the gaps in governmental provisioning. Taken together, these policies signaled to the citizenry a crucial transition in government function; no longer a service provider, the Chinese government instead became a coordinator of services (Chan and Lei 2017; Teets 2012).

Another important shift accompanying social service contracting was the use of domestic, not international, financing for the procurement of services. This change had significant implications for the HIV sector given that up until the mid-2000s, most HIV initiatives had been funded by international donors. As this international funding gradually dwindled, the Chinese government took on more of the financial responsibility for prevention and control. In 2001, the central government invested CNY 100 million (USD 14.5 million) into HIV initiatives, which increased to CNY 1.6 billion (USD 232 million) by 2010 (Wu et al. 2011). It also created a social mobilization fund designed to support social organizations to carry out HIV activities; in 2010–11, this fund distributed CNY 10 million (USD 1.45 million) across seventy-three organizations in the country to implement care, prevention, and capacity-building initiatives (MHPRC 2012).[3] This transition from international to domestic financing may explain why social service contracting, as a government-funded service provision, did not gain serious traction in the HIV sector until the mid- to late 2000s, after the decline of international HIV support.

The departure of the Global Fund from China in 2013–14 left a discernible imprint on HIV groups in the country, partly because it came on the heels of that wider exodus of international donors.[4] With fewer funders and less funding, the number of HIV-related groups was estimated to have dropped by more than two-thirds (Health Policy Project 2016), plunging many HIV organizations into financial precarity. By 2013, key donors, such as the Clinton Foundation, the UK Department for International Development, Australian Aid, and the Ford Foundation, among others, all either left the country or redirected their programmatic focus elsewhere. The Bill and Melinda Gates Foundation concluded its major HIV program in 2013.[5] In short, international donors could no longer be counted on to sustain Chinese organizations as they once had.

This shifting funding landscape galvanized social service contracting in the HIV sector. To fully appreciate the effects, we first need to understand the legacy of Global Fund programs in China, as the Global Fund was one of the most important donors to HIV programs in the country. Since its first HIV/AIDS grant was awarded to China in 2004, the global health donor contributed more than USD 300 million to HIV-related work alone (Global Fund 2020). This money went toward providing ART to people living with HIV, supporting targeted interventions for key populations, and, perhaps most significantly, strengthening the participation of community-based organizations in the HIV sector. Most of the grants earmarked a certain percentage of the budget to be distributed to these organizations to boost their impacts as HIV responders. For example, round 6 of the Global Fund's HIV grant was designed, specifically, to mobilize civil society organizations to scale up HIV prevention and control.

To say that the Global Fund played an important role in China's HIV landscape would be an understatement, and not just because of the size and scale of its financial contributions. Its legacy has been felt at much deeper, structural levels. For one, the Global Fund's support of community-based organizations allowed these organizations to showcase their abilities to reach marginalized populations, such as MSM.[6] They became an asset not only to donors like the Health Fund and ACF but also to government agencies like the Chinese CDC. CDC officials' recognition of community organizations as potential partners grew slowly but surely over time, leading to an interdependence that is now pivotal to the sustainability of these organizations. Because the

Global Fund, even while invested in China, did not operate in-country, its money was channeled to an appointed principal recipient (PR) who managed the grant and oversaw the distribution of funding on the ground. That PR was the Chinese CDC. Since community-based organizations working with MSM benefited substantially from the Global Fund and other international donors, it became critically important for them to maintain cordial relations with the Chinese CDC.

Given the size and longevity of the Global Fund's investment in HIV work in China, any disruption to the Global Fund's grants was guaranteed to have devastating effects on HIV groups, as I witnessed during the course of my fieldwork. In May 2010, a Chinese NGO leader sent a letter to the Global Fund Secretariat complaining that the Chinese CDC, as the PR of the grant, had failed to allocate the requisite percentage of the program budget earmarked for civil society organizations (Jingjing 2013). Following a series of unsuccessful talks, and after an external assessment of China's programs, the Global Fund temporarily suspended its HIV/AIDS grants to the country in October 2010 and, in May 2011, froze funding to almost all of its grants, including those related to tuberculosis and malaria, citing misuse of funds and lack of civil society participation (LaFraniere 2011). Unfortunately, the allegations in China had come on the heels of wider reports of mismanagement of Global Fund money elsewhere, all of which severely damaged the Global Fund's reputation and led its leaders to make internal changes in its grants administration (Clinton and Sridhar 2017a).

By late May 2011, the Chinese government negotiated an agreement to resume Global Fund grants. For their part, Chinese officials agreed to ensure more civil society participation and improve their bookkeeping and accounting measures. By that time, however, the effects of the freeze had already reverberated across China's HIV sector, forcing many organizations to shut their doors permanently.[7] Many of the groups that previously received Global Fund money were legally unregistered (Hildebrandt 2011), and the freeze put them in an even more precarious position, politically as well as economically. I happened to be in the middle of my fieldwork at that time, and I vividly recall the panic that ensued in the wake of the freeze as donors and community leaders alike scrambled to minimize the repercussions from this event. The reactions among those working in the HIV sector were mixed. For some, the freeze was akin to cutting off their lifeline. "Let's be honest," one NGO leader had said. "It's about the money, but without the money, how can we do our work, how can we survive?" And yet, others appeared to welcome the Global Fund's potential departure, particularly those who disliked having to cooperate with the Chinese CDC to access Global Fund resources.

* * * * *

Having outlined the Global Fund's legacy in China, let me now return to how the Global Fund's departure, and that of other donors, advanced social service contracting in China's HIV sector. Thanks to efforts by the Global Fund and others in advocating for the greater participation of civil society organizations in HIV prevention and control, Chinese CDC officials were aware of these organizations' advantages when it came to reaching marginalized populations. As HIV testing among MSM gained traction as a public health strategy, the Chinese CDC began to outsource testing activities, and other interventions, to community-based organizations. It is worth recalling that social service contracting intended to improve cost-efficiency in government operations was already a common practice in other sectors by this time, and its adoption into the HIV sector aligned neatly with widespread endeavors to maximize value for money in public health financing.

In 2008, the Nanjing CDC piloted a project in which it outsourced two of its key services to community-based organizations: testing MSM for HIV and providing care and support to people living with HIV (Yan et al. 2014). Adopting a cash-on-delivery approach whereby payments were distributed upon the completion or meeting of performance targets (similar to the Health Fund's performance-based financing), a study assessing the results of this experiment found that HIV testing and diagnosis rates among MSM increased, as did the rates of early detection of HIV cases and better linkages between detected cases and clinical care, when the work was carried out by community-based organizations. Furthermore, outsourcing these tasks to MSM groups proved to be more cost-effective. The unit cost per HIV case detection by community-based organizations was forty-seven times lower than that by government health facilities (Yan et al. 2014). In other words, community-based organizations identified more HIV-positive MSM at a much lower cost. By 2010, as interest in and the benefits of social service contracting spread, similar arrangements started to appear among CDC agencies in Yunnan, Guangxi, and Shanghai (see Jagusztyn 2012).

HOW A SOCIAL SERVICE CONTRACT PLAYS OUT

Many of the organizations I came to know through ACF and the Health Fund were involved in similar types of activities, either directly testing MSM with rapid HIV tests or recruiting and referring men to the Chinese CDC to get tested, depending on their contracts. For instance, Ah Du, the director of one community-based organization in central China, described its arrangement:

> Our provincial CDC asked us to help them recruit MSM for testing. It cost them about CNY 1,000 (USD 145) each trip to go to gay bars and test these men; their method wasn't cost-effective, and it was cheaper to go through us. The last time they came to us, we organized a training workshop and advertised it on multiple MSM forums online. The CDC administered testing on-site at the event, and collected about 400 tests from this activity. We received CNY 8,000 (USD 1,161).

Ah Du emphasized the cost-effectiveness of administering HIV testing through his organization as compared to the efforts of the Chinese CDC. "They only ever succeeded in getting a few tests," he commented of the CDC's mobilization endeavors, contrasting their dismal number with the hundreds of men made available to the CDC for testing through his organization's reach. A similar narrative was offered by Xiao Xiao, the director of a community-based organization in central China:

> The CDC paid our organization CNY 25,000 (USD 3,629) every six months to organize one training workshop per month targeting MSM. We were given targets to reach 2,000 men and collect 400 HIV tests in addition to meeting other countable services such as condoms distributed. We earned up to CNY 1,062 (USD 154) per person tested and diagnosed for HIV. The CDC recently started accepting results from our rapid HIV testing; this means that instead of the CDC administering on-site testing at different locales, they just accept our rapid HIV tests. They no longer accompany us to do testing because it costs too much for them.

In his case, Xiao Xiao's organization had cultivated enough trust, or *guanxi,* with the local Chinese CDC for the latter to accept rapid HIV tests administered by his organization in lieu of the preliminary HIV test conventionally conducted by the CDC. This step meant that rather than men getting a rapid HIV test by the organization, then a preliminary test by the CDC, and later a confirmation test by the CDC if the preliminary screening was positive (required to be eligible for free ART), MSM were now able to take a rapid HIV test given by Xiao Xiao's organization and then proceed directly to a confirmation test if and as needed, thereby eliminating the preliminary test altogether. This abridged process, Xiao Xiao emphasized, made scaling up MSM testing more cost-effective for the Chinese CDC, in terms of both its time and its labor, and it ensured that more men were tested. Community-based organizations, therefore, played a critical role in these arrangements, not only by carrying out tasks for the Chinese CDC but also by providing care in the form of testing, diagnosis, and counseling to MSM. The relevance of community-based organizations in China reflects a global trend in which NGOs and other social actors take on increasingly varied and complex roles (Fisher 1997; Bernal and Grewal 2014; Leve and Karim 2001).

Community-based organizations have long interested anthropologists. Lamia Karim (2011) suggested that NGOs operate as a "shadow state" that provides key services to citizens but also ushers in neoliberal agendas. In her study of microfinance NGOs in Bangladesh, she showed how these organizations, rather than being apolitical and neutral, were deeply entrenched in political networks, sometimes masking their politics behind a humanitarian ethos. But in other scenarios, as Peter Redfield (2013) illustrated in his work with Médicins Sans Frontières (MSF), NGOs are susceptible to the tensions of wider humanitarian systems and politics. In global health, these tensions are especially acute given the significant amount of resources being channeled to and from NGOs, which have the power to determine where and how those resources are used (McCoy, Chand, and Sridhar 2009; Ravishankar et al. 2009). NGOs, like those who fund them, therefore cannot be viewed simply as straightforward service providers; rather, they are pivotal intermediaries in delivering care and also in configuring what care does and does not entail.

I first started hearing about social service contracting early on in my fieldwork, as more and more CDC agencies began utilizing the practice in their provinces and cities. In principle, social service contracting seemed to promise a win-win scenario for all actors involved by financially sustaining community-based organizations while allowing government agencies—in this case, the Chinese CDC—to improve "their" service provision by way of community-based organizations. Both ACF and the Health Fund actively encouraged their grantees to seek out these opportunities, touting them as a potential palliative to diminishing international resources. I once heard Jonah caution those working in community-based organizations, "We are not going to support you forever, and you need to be able to keep providing services for the community once a project ends." His reproach served as an ominous reminder that international funding is never guaranteed.

The Health Fund initiated a series of pilot projects across select cities to test out the practice, and as a way of promoting it to the Chinese CDC. As a result, many people credited the Health Fund for advancing social service contracting in China's HIV sector. Zhang Li even suggested that social service contracting may end up being one of the Health Fund's most enduring legacies, and not just because many of the contracts were developed to include performance-based financing structures utilized in the Health Fund's program.

In what remains of this chapter, I describe how social service contracting has rearranged the kinds of services and forms of care community-based organizations provide to MSM. I show how endeavors to scale up testing among MSM increasingly came to be shaped by the demand for performance targets and the need for performance incentives to sustain these organizations. I do not suggest that performance targets and incentives are the only reason MSM groups carried out testing and diagnosis; on the contrary, many of the groups I met over the course of my research exhibited a fierce commitment to reducing HIV transmission in their communities and caring for MSM. Instead, I am interested in how structures like social service contracting directed how prevention and care were implemented. As Zhang Li once said to me, "a lot of organizations rely on MSM testing simply to survive, as a livelihood; and in the government, it is all about testing."

Social service contracting in the HIV sector at the time of my research was primarily used for MSM testing and diagnosis. Many community-based organizations involved with these arrangements reorganized their activities to meet the performance metrics because only by meeting targets would they remain attractive to the CDC. This focus marginalized other forms of prevention and care that could have been equally, if not more, important to reducing HIV in China's MSM community.

I start by presenting a Request for Proposals (RFP) released by a provincial CDC as an example of how public tenders look. I then present two examples of community-based organizations involved in social service contracting with their local CDCs and describe their activities, along with the strategies they used to meet performance goals. I illustrate how both social service contracting and the performance metrics that characterize them have reshaped the landscape of HIV prevention and care.

A Request for Proposals (RFP)

In 2014, I came across a public RFP published on the website of a provincial CDC in Southwest China seeking to procure HIV testing and other services from community-based organizations. I was alerted to this announcement by Zhang Li, who by that time had left her position at a public health agency and taken on a new role as the regional director of an NGO. She planned to submit a proposal to this RFP on behalf of Huang Yueliang (hereinafter referred to as Yellow Moon), a small, unregistered organization serving MSM.[8] To be eligible, organizations were required to be legally established, though not registered, in the city where the provincial CDC was based and to maintain an independent financial system capable of processing program funds. Since Yellow Moon lacked such an independent financial system, a fairly common scenario for many community organizations, it opted to go through Zhang Li's NGO as a sponsoring agency.

This particular RFP was one of the first "public" announcements inviting organizations to submit proposals to the Chinese CDC of which I was aware. Most of the contracts I came across were negotiated internally between CDC agencies and select community-based organizations, rather than undergoing an open tender. This public announcement seemed, at least on the surface, to mark a turning point to a more open and transparent process, one more in line with the guidelines prescribed since the late 1990s, and diverging from more *guanxi*-oriented arrangements characterizing earlier iterations of these contracts. In this particular RFP, three separate projects were listed for bidding.

The first project, "HIV Testing Mobilization for Men Who Have Sex with Men," outlined two primary goals: to reduce high-risk behaviors related to the spread of STIs in MSM and to increase HIV testing, counseling, and notification of results to reduce the number of men lost after an HIV screening. To meet these objectives, applicants were required to carry out a range of activities, including, but not limited to, administering HIV testing and counseling with the use of rapid HIV tests, providing pre- and posttest counseling to newly diagnosed HIV-positive men, and ensuring the completion of any and all paperwork for on-site activities, such as the collection of personal data, to minimize loss to follow-up. Testing was restricted to men who had had same-sex sexual contact but had not received an HIV test in the past three months, presumably to prevent the problem of "repeat testers" that had beset the Health Fund's program. To avert any potential deception, the RFP limited testing to no more than six thousand MSM citywide across all awarded grantees, budgeted at CNY 50 (USD 7) per HIV test and CNY 600 (USD 87) per new HIV case detected, subject to verification by the Chinese CDC. The higher rates for identifying new HIV cases, as in the Health Fund's program, were meant to incentivize groups to work harder to identify more new infections.

The second project, "Community Care Service Program for HIV Cases," supported treatment and counseling services for people living with HIV. It sought to ensure timely follow-up care and support to patients as part of maintaining their physical and emotional well-being. These services extended to regular clinical testing (CD4, tuberculosis, viral loads), ART adherence, HIV/STI health counseling and prevention, psychological counseling and family care, and HIV testing for all sexual partners to promote behavioral change and reduce HIV transmission. Grantees were expected to prepare individual case files for each patient, which had to include written session notes on the topics discussed and any actionable items taken by the grantee. For example, outputs might include steps taken to help the client overcome psychological problems (such as a referral to a counselor), or improving ART adherence, or aiding the client to undergo clinical testing (such as CD4). Because the activities in this project were to be administered over a longer period of time, payments were made per "series" of services, which included an annual HIV test of the negative-status partner, a tuberculosis screening of people living with HIV, a CD4 test and two follow-up visits for HIV-positive persons, and two CD4 tests and four follow-up visits for AIDS patients. For each service package completed, grantees were paid CNY 200 (USD 29).

The third and final project, "Quality HIV Intervention Program for Colleges," targeted college students in and around local universities in the city, but especially male students having sex with other men, for HIV-related risk behavior interventions. This project called on grantees to "innovate intervention models" by using peer-education methods that promoted behavioral change, with an explicit aim to mobilize male students for HIV testing and counseling. The guidelines remained relatively vague, requiring only that grantees submit a feasibility analysis detailing the needs of their demographic alongside measurable goals and an evaluation plan that would be used to assess the effectiveness of the activities. Of all the projects listed, this one offered the most flexibility in terms of outreach activities, only stipulating that the end goal should be to test and treat male youths who have sex with men.

For each of the listed projects, little if any guidance as to how the applicants should go about meeting the targets was provided, giving them the flexibility to choose the "how" of their activities so long as the "what" of them, meaning performance targets, was met. Unlike more conventional donor projects where applicants budgeted for inputs such as administrative costs, educational materials, condoms, and other items in advance, the CDC in this case had adopted performance-based financing mechanisms and intended only to pay awardees for the outputs delivered.

The versatility enabled by performance-based financing systems is appealing to donors because it allows them (or, in this case, it allowed the Chinese CDC) a hands-off approach in which what are counted, and paid for, are the desired results (Eichler, Levine, and PBI 2009). This kind of flexibility should, ideally, motivate service providers (or community-based organizations) to innovate to compete and, in doing so, should ensure better health outcomes for patients/clients. The social service contracting arrangements described by Ah Du and Xiao Xiao earlier illustrate the potential advantages of this process perfectly: the CDC (donor) is able to reach its testing targets while providing little oversight and thus investing minimal labor as well as mitigating operational expenses.

Anthropologists, however, caution against such optimism, arguing that prioritizing financial outcomes does not always lead to improved health outcomes. Instead, they suggest that conflating financial and health outcomes often exacerbates the very health inequities that health interventions are intended to address (see, e.g., Biehl and Petryna 2013; Crane 2013; Fan and Uretsky 2017). What counts, and according to whom, as better health outcomes for patients is a question that many anthropologists have been quick to pose. As I show in the subsequent sections, community-based organizations implement different activities to reach and test MSM; yet, the pressure to meet performance targets limits their ability to provide longer-term care to their beneficiaries.

Submitting a Proposal: The Importance of Performance Targets

The demand for numbers in social service contracts, as seen in the aforementioned RFP, gradually reoriented how community-based organizations carried out their work. The decline of international HIV support led to more than a crisis of money; it provoked a crisis of conscience in relation to how organizations performed HIV services and cared for their communities. In my fieldwork, I consistently heard complaints, voiced by leaders of community-based organizations, about their groups being used as puppets by the CDC and donors. These sentiments underscored the ambivalent relationships that community-based organizations had with the Chinese CDC; they also revealed the precarity of those groups, which too often had to "adjust their mission[s] or modify their work in order to get funding," as one community activist said to me.[9] For organizations, such as Yellow Moon, that were unregistered and relied heavily on international donors, and for which social service contracting and other forms of governmental support were fundamental to organizational sustainability, meeting performance targets mattered. Failure to do so was to sacrifice opportunities for earning contracts in the future.

I came to know Yellow Moon through my work with ACF, as it was a grantee of ACF's projects. When I spent some time shadowing Zhang Li in her new position in Southwest China, I got the chance to know the organization more intimately. As an unregistered youth organization providing sexual health services to its community, staff and volunteers of Yellow Moon were well aware of their capacity to reach and test large numbers of MSM. They cultivated, over the years, a strong network of college-aged students and young adults, especially MSM, as a result of director Wei Wei's involvement in the gay community as a self-identified "gay" (in English) man. Yellow Moon sustained this network, as well as its service provision, by relying on a handful of staff and a revolving door of volunteers who left just as quickly as they could be replaced. As such, Yellow Moon was representative of the majority of HIV and MSM groups supported and eventually left behind by international donors. Numbers, and delivering "good" numbers, in this context, played an increasingly important role in guiding the organization's social service contracting arrangements.

Taking stock of its capacity, Yellow Moon's leaders decided to apply for two out of the three projects listed in the aforementioned RFP: the first (HIV testing among MSM) and the third (HIV interventions in college-aged youths). In preparing its application, Yellow Moon staff were required to develop budget proposals outlining their expected targets for HIV testing and detection, which would fit the payment rates set out in the RFP. After much internal discussion and conversation with Zhang Li, whose organization acted as the sponsoring agency, Yellow Moon staff and volunteers decided to propose a modest budget to test eight hundred MSM (paid at CNY 50, or USD 7, per test) and to detect thirty new HIV cases (paid at CNY 600 each, or USD 87) for the first project. I recall being in the room when this decision was made and wondering how anyone could know in advance the number of HIV-positive men a project would discover.

Logically, Zhang Li explained to me, these predictions are derived from existing HIV data provided by the Chinese CDC. If CDC data showed, for example, that 7 percent of MSM in a city are HIV-positive, then applicants in that city know to propose a target of HIV-positive cases that is fewer than that number. The CDC data offered both a gauge for estimating potential cases and a range within which HIV cases could be situated; any number above or too far below was likely to imply inaccuracy at best or deception at worst. As Wei Wei explained, "in our proposal, we say that we will detect thirty new HIV cases out of the total eight hundred HIV tests we plan to carry out, but that number [thirty] is only three percent of the total number of tests we are conducting [eight hundred]. . . . It is unlikely we will not reach that number . . . [because] if we do not, then we are probably testing the wrong population [i.e., individuals who are not MSM]." According to Wei Wei, setting a target of 3 percent "ensures that we are testing the right population."[10]

Wei Wei's interpretation of data and performance targets indicated to me that he had a clear understanding of the stakes involved in meeting performance goals within social service contracts. Meeting these safe-guarded, to some degree, an organization's economic future, while not meeting performance goals jeopardized prospective contracts. Casey Miller (2016) has described how the Chinese CDC ranked NGOs ac-cording to the number of tests (among MSM) each administered and the number of positive HIV cases each detected, allocating more lucra-tive contracts to those that had higher numbers. Performance targets act as proof of work and verify an organization's credibility. By submit-ting the "right" numbers—those that aligned to the CDC data—Yellow Moon would show that it was able to reach "real" MSM and therefore protect itself against accusations of cheating or duplicity. Zhang Li once recounted to me how the Health Fund came to discover deception in its program: "We knew that a city had 10 percent HIV prevalence among MSM, and then an organization came along and claims to have tested 100 men but did not identify any HIV-positive cases; then how is that possible? It must be that the group is either deliberately manipulating their numbers or they are simply not testing real MSM." Providing the CDC with the numbers they expected became even more important following the rumors of deception and corruption in the Health Fund's program.

The difficulties transpiring in the Health Fund's program undoubt-edly shaped the CDC's decision to use performance-based financing in social service contracts, reinforcing the belief that numbers are best suited to measuring accountability. The presumption about numbers, of course, is that they tell the truth, or rather *a* truth, in a way that is apolitical, objective, and neutral (Porter 1995). In such a world, an or-ganization that does not return the "right" numbers might signal to the funder that it is lying, or worse yet, that it does not possess the capacity or skill to reach "real" MSM and meet performance targets. Figures too high suggest that an organization is engaging in deceptive practices to manufacture numbers. In either case, to not meet performance targets places at risk an organization's reputation and its potential to attain additional contracts. Numbers in the form of targets, then, serve as "devices for self-monitoring" (Ferguson and Gupta 2002, 987) insofar as they reinforce surveillance and discipline of and by community-based organizations. The right numbers also allow the Chinese CDC to justify its health spending decisions using arguments that it is maximizing value for money.

For community-based organizations participating in this system, the task of "performing data is just part of the job" (Erikson 2012, 374). At play here is not so much the accuracy of the numbers as what the numbers do and how they organize health priorities. In her ethnographic study of the Chinese public health system, Katherine Mason (2016) distinguished between the production of "correct" data and "true" data within the Chinese CDC; "correct" data were structured by *guanxi* (personal relations) for the purposes of preserving those networks but often led to misreporting, whereas "true" data more adequately captured on-the-ground circumstances but risked disrupting the social ties that were crucial to getting things done. These sorts of negotiations, argued Anthony Spires (2011), were a necessary practice by local government agencies that needed to gain "political credit" from their superiors in upper administrations of government. Spires provided an example whereby the head of a provincial party committee informed hospital administrators that they would be fired if they "reported" any cases of avian flu, not if they "had" any cases, drawing a careful distinction between the reality of public health data and the documentation of it. Even if CDC numbers are flawed or black boxed or kept secret, as Mason illustrated, they nonetheless do performative work to hold grantees accountable and reinforce the authority of CDC data, something Wei Wei and other leaders of community-based organizations understood well.[11]

The pressure to meet performance targets led some organizations to sacrifice quality to deliver quantity. A 2014 study conducted for USAID examined the rollout of social service contracting in the HIV sector in select provinces; it found that in some places, local health authorities insisted that organizations to whom they contract out testing "persuade" people to get tested in order to scale up numbers, a practice that stood in contradistinction to the preference of these organizations to carry out testing only after individuals were convinced of the benefits and responsibilities of getting tested (Jagusztyn 2014). This study illustrates the untenable position in which many organizations now find themselves; and yet, it also shows how bureaucratic pressures from above profoundly shape the way organizations carry out their work.

Internet-Based Outreach: The Case of Red Love

For Hong Ai (hereinafter referred to as Red Love), a youth organization promoting sexual health among MSM in southeastern China, digital and social media platforms played a key role in their testing and counseling strategies. The composition of Red Love staff and volunteers largely reflected the demography they sought to serve: youths under the age of thirty and savvy in the use of digital technologies. The organization utilized popular Chinese platforms, such as WeChat, QQ, and SMS, to advertise its HIV testing services along with more traditional activities like telephone hotlines, peer-education advocacy, care and support groups, and psychological counseling. As Xiao Li, the young and dynamic director of Red Love, said, "our organization takes advantage of new media such as WeChat, 400 hotline, and text messaging to multiple recipients to promote HIV/VCT-related information. . . . At the same time, outreach intervention measures are adopted to increase population coverage so as not to target the same demographic repeatedly."

The last part of this statement was a nod to the organization's ability to identify "new" (*faxianzhe*) and not only existing HIV cases (*ganranzhe*), as required by the CDC. This preference for "new" cases was intended to discourage repeat testing practices. Xiao Li (who has identified as tongzhi and tongxinglian but remained, until recently, in a long-term relationship with his girlfriend) detailed another mechanism put into place by the CDC to protect against deception: "Our CDC only distributes payments if the person [getting tested] goes through the entire process of confirming an HIV diagnosis, from preliminary HIV screening to CD4 testing." This means that a person who initially elicits a positive test (if administered via rapid HIV test by the organization, for example) must undergo confirmation testing at the Chinese CDC to verify the HIV diagnosis. Because confirmation HIV tests are administered by the Chinese CDC, an HIV diagnosis is only the first step in a series of other clinical tests that the CDC administers to persons confirmed to be HIV-positive, including a CD4 test to monitor a person's CD4 count. Only if an individual completes all the clinical tests administered by the CDC after an HIV diagnosis does the CDC count the person as part of the performance targets and issue payment to the organization. This process is required by the CDC to monitor that the organization has completed its tasks in getting a person tested and an HIV diagnosis confirmed by the CDC, rather than relying on the organization to self-report the number of HIV-positive cases it identified. In the case that an individual does not go through the process from start to finish (e.g., confirming an HIV diagnosis at the Chinese CDC but not going through CD4 testing), the HIV tests and the HIV cases can be counted toward meeting the performance targets but cannot be submitted for payment.[12] This practice protects the Chinese CDC from making payments for incomplete tasks thus lowering its overall health spending.

Xiao Li credited its leveraging of digital technologies with enabling Red Love to consistently meet the targets assigned by its provincial CDC. In its particular case, social service agreements were negotiated internally between Red Love and that CDC, without a public bidding process. Xiao Li attributed this arrangement to the strong *guanxi,* and trust, built up with the local CDC leaders over the years, a relationship no doubt strengthened by Red Love's consistent success in delivering outputs. In one contract, for example, the CDC assigned Red Love the following targets: 4,000 MSM to be tested for HIV (paid at CNY 150, or USD 23, per test) and 175 men to be "detected positive" (paid at CNY 600, or USD 91, per case). Red Love met both easily. The CDC also gave the organization specific metrics to expand "coverage" of MSM using digital technologies: two thousand MSM to be reached by QQ, two thousand by text messaging (SMS), and fifteen hundred by WeChat. Xiao Li admitted that he knew meeting these targets would be challenging for the organization's core staff, so Red Love hired additional part-time staff to assist with MSM testing to meet the targets.[13]

Red Love employed a combination of in-person and online strategies to mobilize MSM for testing. Digital and social media platforms were leveraged to advertise its HIV testing services and direct men to get tested at any of its sites and events, and then again to simplify and expedite follow-up communications. For instance, applications like QQ and WeChat were harnessed to deliver pre- and posttest consultations conducted entirely online. To this end, Red Love created a WeChat page that allowed visitors to schedule testing appointments directly through the app. In a typical week, and as part of its regular services, Red Love offered rapid HIV testing (oral and finger prick) every day at its offices. On select days (Tuesdays, Wednesdays, and Thursdays), these services were made available at the local CDC office. Additionally, Red Love organized large-scale activities geared toward HIV testing at least three to four times a week, mainly on weekends. It advertised free condoms and lubricants online and distributed these to promote safe sexual practices.

Red Love was one of many organizations adopting internet-based strategies to do outreach; its digital savvy enabled it to innovate ways to expand MSM testing. In 2014, for instance, nearly 60 percent of the four thousand HIV tests Red Love carried out among MSM were the result of WeChat-based recruitment efforts. Huang et al. found in a public health study in 2012 that the number of men recruited for testing from online platforms far exceeded the number of men recruited through physical venues. This study, along with several others, confirmed that an increasing number of MSM, especially younger MSM, are using online platforms and social media apps to communicate with one another and to seek out HIV services (China-Gates Foundation HIV Prevention Cooperation Program 2013; Feng, Wu, and Detels 2010; Han et al. 2016).

Digital technologies are not only useful for outreach; they are also one of the ways by which MSM are "made up," a process that has been pivotal to mobilizing MSM in China to get tested voluntarily. Not incidentally, "making up" MSM is also well suited to meeting performance targets. Scholars have long attended to how media—print, mass, social—act as powerful forces in shaping the way people come to think about community, sexuality, and health. For many Chinese MSM at the time of my fieldwork, the internet was both a site to meet other men and a source of information for thinking of oneself as tongzhi or any other same-sex desiring identity, furnishing men with positive templates for same-sex living (Sun, Farrer, and Choi 2006). The internet provided many "a-ha" moments for Chinese MSM, not unlike those described by Tom Boellstorff (2003), who found that it was not uncommon for the Indonesians with whom he worked to come to think of themselves as *gay* or *lesbi* through encounters with mainstream media—or, as I described in chapter 2, through *ziworentong* workshops.

Indeed, the power of online platforms to do things is evidenced by

Red Love's success in leveraging digital technologies to get MSM tested. Xiao Li estimated that testing alone produced nearly 30 percent of the organization's total budget. Red Love increased the cost of its rapid HIV testing services from CNY 30 (USD 4) to CNY 100 (USD 15) in the four years leading up to 2011, and still it was able to meet the testing targets set by its Chinese CDC.

Despite the success of Red Love's endeavors, Xiao Li nonetheless expressed doubts related to the effects of HIV testing interventions. He lamented that testing had become a quick and convenient technical intervention yet did not necessarily encourage men to change their risky behaviors. Xiao Li and other leaders of community-based organizations questioned the utility of testing as practiced in this manner, as a method that offered short-term returns, such as epidemiological data, but did not address longer-term challenges that led men to get infected in the first place. Xiao Li admitted that in Red Love's testing initiatives, the organization did little in terms of posttesting follow-up for men testing negative other than providing information about transmission. "If quantitative indicators are imposed, then you will chase after those indicators; then, your goal becomes *shuliang* [quantity], not *zhiliang* [quality]," he bemoaned. His statement captures well the drawbacks of social service contracting but also of performance-based financing.

Same-Sex Communal Spaces: The Case of Blue Heart

While occupying digital and social media spaces was key to Red Love's success in fulfilling social service contracts, Blue Heart (introduced in chapter 2) directed its efforts toward reaching MSM in more traditionally communal same-sex areas, such as bathhouses. Blue Heart was a small MSM group located in northeastern China, staffed by two individuals since its inception: director Bao Hua and longtime volunteer Xiao Qi. The organization operated in a "second-tier" (smaller, less dense) city where stigma attached to MSM was particularly acute, as was social pressure for Chinese men to marry heterosexually. Xiao Qi, for example, self-identifies as a tongzhi yet had, for years and only until recently, assumed he was getting married; his long-term boyfriend remained married throughout their relationship. Bao Hua, in contrast, identifies publicly as tongzhi and has remained in a same-sex relationship for the past decade. Nevertheless, for many MSM in the city, same-sex sexual experiences continued to be hidden, relegated to private spaces like bathhouses, well-known gathering spots for men seeking other men. In this case, the city had a bathhouse that hosted a mixture of local and out-of-town men.

Blue Heart's social service arrangement with its local CDC diverged from that of Yellow Moon and the public bidding process and Red Love's activity-specific metrics. For the past five years, the CDC provided CNY 16,500 (USD 2,500) to Blue Heart annually to test four hundred MSM in its city. In its case, there was no monetary distinction made between testing and diagnosing MSM. Bao Hua admitted that they came late to the social service game since they struggled to develop good *guanxi* with their CDC but had since improved their relations and the CDC by then came to them directly. The local CDC maintained minimal oversight of Blue Heart's activities, leaving it up to the organization to determine how best to test MSM, so long as the performance targets were met. According to Bao Hua, Blue Heart had never not met these targets.

Bathhouses are productive sites for HIV testing because they reinforce sociality and community among their members, making them a space where MSM are readily available for testing. These same-sex spaces, not unlike the virtual spaces accessed through digital technologies, mediate relationships between the self and the community. Men who go into such spaces do so as part of a community of men seeking other men, and they reinforce understandings of themselves as men seeking other men by entering into these spaces, regardless of their lifestyles and marital statuses outside of these spaces.

Blue Heart's commitment to basing its testing recruitment and outreach efforts in and around a bathhouse in the city was informed by a number of factors, not least of which was the size and demographic of that city. Many of the men they sought were older, unlikely to be online, and publicly in relationships with women. These men did not always perceive HIV to be an imminent risk, Bao Hua explained: "In a city like ours, men see *aizibing* [HIV and AIDS] as something that happens in big cities, not as something that could affect them." Thus Blue Heart opted to set up HIV testing stations inside the local bathhouse. Xiao Qi explained that testing areas were assembled in a semiprivate room on the second floor of the bathhouse. There, men could and did come in for quick pre- and posttest consultations and rapid HIV tests. Bao Hua stressed that the consultations were an important part of the rapid testing process, and the tests were always administered one-on-one so as to protect the confidentiality of those being tested. Having developed good *guanxi* with the bathhouse owner, Bao Hua and the Blue Heart volunteers were able to administer testing services inside the bathhouse once every two weeks.

Their strategy proved, for the most part, effective; Xiao Qi claimed that inside the bathhouse was where Blue Heart found the most HIV-positive cases. According to Bao Hua, "one year we probably tested about three hundred men, and forty-two of them turned out to be HIV-positive," roughly 14 percent of the men tested. He attributed the high rates of HIV in the bathhouse to the notion that "men who go to the bathhouse are the ones that do not admit to their [same-sex] sexual identity." Xiao Qi echoed this sentiment, noting that "men like [the bathhouse] because it is dark and promises anonymity, and since they go there for sex, not for friendships or relationships, there is little risk of them getting outed." To be sure, he acknowledged that many of the men who tested positive in the bathhouse were, in fact, married. Furthermore, condoms were rarely if ever used at the bathhouse, which drove up HIV rates among men seeking sexual partners in these same-sex spaces (Dong et al. 2019).

I asked Xiao Qi what happened after they administered rapid testing in the bathhouse: "If men test HIV-positive, do they go back downstairs and continue having sex?" In response, he admitted that he did not know the answer, because it was infeasible for Blue Heart volunteers to venture downstairs after each HIV test and monitor the activities of the men. Blue Heart's strategy relied heavily on the men getting tested to follow up on their rapid HIV test at a later date in Blue Heart's offices, but, as Xiao Qi recognized, not all of the men tested did so. At best, he told me, one of their more daring volunteers sometimes goes downstairs to hand out condoms to the men to encourage safe sexual practices.

I couldn't help but wonder what happens to the men not captured in the HIV-positive count, or to the men who tested positive with the rapid HIV test but never followed up to confirm their diagnoses, or who returned to their same-sex sexual activities inside and outside the bathhouse. Still yet, what of the out-of-town men who test HIV-positive? There is little doubt that scaling up HIV testing among Chinese MSM has saved countless lives, many of those lives belonging to the men I met during fieldwork. Recent studies show an increase in the annual testing rate among these men, from 16.6 percent in 2009 to 58.6 percent in 2011 (Chow et al. 2013; see also Zou et al. 2012). At the same time, I am made aware of how the demand for metrics and performance incentives made it so that only HIV testing and the steps leading up to the test mattered in providing care to MSM. I do not mean to say that community-based organizations only care about meeting performance targets; rather, I argue that they cannot afford not to care about these metrics, and these are frequently prioritized at the expense of providing longer-term, comprehensive care.

CONCLUSION

In summer 2015, I returned to China to conduct supplementary fieldwork for my research project. One night, at a reunion dinner with some of the leaders of community-based organizations with whom I had worked during my earlier fieldwork, the conversation turned to advocating for MSM issues other than HIV and testing. Some of the men in the room complained that any discussion of the needs of MSM seemed to revolve only around HIV. Many worried about the narrow focus on testing MSM. One of the men explained, "As a 'gay' man, HIV is not always a priority for us; there are other things we think about as 'gay' men, and we don't want HIV to be the thing that defines us." His sentiments were echoed by another, who said, "Everywhere I go, it is testing and HIV, testing and HIV, as if this is the only thing that is important in the gay community." "HIV is *zhongyao* [important], but not a *zhongdian* [focal point]," added another of the men present.

These comments reflect the discontent among leaders of community-based organizations and activists working on HIV issues toward practices like social service contracting and the use of performance metrics to scale up MSM testing over the years. Indeed, social service contracting effectively institutionalized into local health systems MSM testing as a core and sometimes sole strategy for controlling the epidemic in China and, certainly, a key approach to addressing HIV in this population. This left community-based organizations with little time or money for advocating for MSM as complex human beings, as diverse in their care needs, as more than bodies to be tested.

As the case studies showed, the use of performance-based financing by the CDC in social service contracts to encourage innovation capable

of improving health outcomes did not always succeed. Instead, the linking of performance targets and incentives to testing metrics constrained
organizations to short-term services like HIV testing and diagnosis
rather than longer-term, and possibly more preventative, interventions.
To be sure, a central component of social service contracting relied on
techniques of counting that translated results into epidemiological data,
for example, how many men are infected, but did not tell us how or
why MSM were contracting HIV in the first place or how they were
responding after an HIV-positive diagnosis. Performance metrics have
reshaped what counts, is thinkable, and is possible in HIV prevention
and care. In reflecting on these processes, I wonder if asking how men
are contracting HIV, or how they might be understanding their HIV
risk, may produce a different approach, and response, to preventing
and controlling the epidemic altogether.

REMAKING COMMUNITIES
OF BELONGING

IN NOVEMBER 2010, shortly after I began my long-term fieldwork, Jonah (director of ACF) invited me to a gathering, or "informal conversation," as he put it, that he had organized for key stakeholders in the HIV sector. The purpose of the meeting was to brainstorm how to better support community-based organizations to carry out their work. Initially slated to be hosted at my small but cozy apartment in Beijing, he later shifted the venue to the offices of the Health Fund, as its staff generously offered up its spacious conference room for the gathering. The composition of the meeting was meant to reflect the diversity of a community ostensibly driven by a collective goal to prevent and control the HIV epidemic. As such, it included members from community-based organizations, international donors, and public health agencies. Particularly noteworthy was the fact that most of the community leaders in the meeting represented organizations serving MSM (rather than sex workers or other HIV- and AIDS-affected populations), a telling sign of the prevalence of MSM and MSM testing in China's public health landscape.

Having just recently arrived and still settling into my field site, I quietly made my way to one edge of the room, from where I observed people around me greet their friends and colleagues. Very quickly, the alliances among those present became visible. To my relief, I spotted Fu Xiao, an HIV activist and one-time ally of Jonah and with whom I was friendly, as he entered the room. Upon seeing me, Fu Xiao headed over. He sat down next to me, and as we chatted, he provided a running commentary of the attendees as they entered the room. At one point, I recognized a colleague and asked, "Is that so and so?" Fu Xiao, perhaps anticipating an introduction, quickly replied, "Yes, but I am not speaking to him because I don't like him." He then called this person a phony, which proved to be a sentiment that many of my interlocutors, throughout my time in the field, would use to describe a vast number of HIV activists and leaders. When Jonah stood up to start the meeting, Fu Xiao leaned over and whispered to me, "I think Jonah is only having this meeting to show himself to be the leader in the community." His suggestion that Jonah had personal motives for hosting the meeting seemed to me yet another way of saying "phony."

Fu Xiao's comment about Jonah, though only an aside whispered to me, betrayed the deepening tensions that permeated the community being represented at that meeting. These tensions, I came to gather, arose in large part from the distinction between *community*-based and *project*-based organizations, that is, those guided by mission (the former) and those motivated by money (the latter). One of the meeting participants, a director of a community-based organization serving MSM, described his struggles to remain community driven rather than project driven in his work, drawing an intentional contrast between taking on projects that advanced his organization's objectives and chasing after projects for money. He detailed his fatigue from constantly searching for funding just to stay afloat while trying to preserve that mission. His exhaustion resonated with Bao Hua, the director of Blue Heart (see chapter 3), who added that his organization recently started to attract external funding, but only after years of going without. These directors' experiences revealed the challenges community-based organizations faced, especially when they remained committed to outreach efforts and providing services out of principle, refusing to be directed by funding alone.

Many of the community activists in the room that day echoed these men's sentiments, and some blamed international donors and public health institutions like the Chinese CDC for the pressures they shouldered to chase after money. Fu Xiao alleged that these pressures had led the tongzhi movement to go "completely off-track," as he put it, alleging that many organizations had become "pawns and proxies" of donors and the Chinese CDC, given that these larger players controlled the flow of financial resources upon which the smaller organizations relied. Fu Xiao questioned how many organizations were actually sustainable at that time, especially among those that strove to remain community driven but whose projects were not HIV testing-centric.

Another community leader in the room asserted that organizations had resorted to "serving the project" *(wei xiangmu fuwu)* rather than their communities.[1]

Those in the room who represented donor organizations and the CDC were quick to respond. They redirected blame onto the smaller organizations, accusing the leaders of these organizations of chasing after money. As one woman chastised, too many grantees were just "following the money and doing whatever projects came up rather than keeping to a focused strategy and goal." She suggested that if and when organizations failed, it was because they prioritized money (project based) over principle (community based), calling into question the integrity of these organizations. Yang Xia, the program officer for the Health Fund, reiterated yet softened the woman's critique by gently advising the organizations' leaders first to determine a clear mission and then to let that mission guide their decisions. "You can always say no to a project [if it doesn't advance the right goals]," she told them.

Yang Xia's comments, although meant to be constructive, were poorly received by the community leaders in the room, setting off a maelstrom of anger. Huang Wei, a long-standing activist and director of a tongzhi group in northwestern China whom I knew to be a vocal critic of international donors, criticized the Health Fund for essentially forcing community-based organizations to "serve the project" to survive. He challenged their authority to set programmatic priorities for a community of which they were not a part and which they did not understand. He argued that just as non-tongzhi could not represent the interests of tongzhi, donors like the Health Fund could not dictate local communities' needs. "We know the community, our needs, and how to implement projects," he asserted. "Why does an outside expert need to come in and tell us how to do our jobs?" His anger swiftly spread to other community leaders in the room. "You [the Health Fund] come into our community and tell us how to do our jobs?" admonished another man present. Fu Xiao added that "it is the community that should be helping the community," making it clear that the Health Fund did not belong.

* * * * *

Huang Wei's, Fu Xiao's, and other community leaders' anger during that meeting underscored a deeper tension at play in the "community," which I use here to mean activists and organizations serving MSM. The tension, as I describe in this chapter, stemmed from a distinction many participants made between "real" *(zhen)* or community-based organizations and "fake" *(jia)* or project-based ones. Indeed, the terms *real* and *fake* were consistently invoked by my interlocutors to distinguish themselves, as real, from others. Real organizations were understood to deliver a wide array of care and support services to MSM. They were driven by "good intentions" and committed to advancing greater social change for MSM. In contrast, fake organizations were understood to be driven by funding and other material benefits.

I focus in this chapter on the distinction between real and fake organizations as it appeared throughout my fieldwork and on the anxieties this distinction provoked within the community of those who worked to reduce HIV transmission among MSM. In this chapter and the next, I start to trace the aftermath of scaling up MSM testing in China. By "aftermath," I do not mean that the intervention has ended; rather, I am interested in understanding how it has unraveled in the communities and lives of those affected by its implementation. I ask, How has HIV testing exacerbated the already present fractures in the community? How has testing evoked reimaginings of belonging across the HIV landscape? By attending to these questions, I provide insights into the social and cultural effects of health interventions like MSM testing. I suggest that these interventions can undermine, rather than empower, a community of activists and organizations committed to MSM advocacy.

THE POLITICS OF EATING AIDS RICE

When distinguishing between community-based and project-based organizations, I came across interlocutors frequently using the phrase *chi aizibing de fan,* or eating AIDS rice. Eating AIDS rice, or consuming from the AIDS rice bowl, implies that a person or, as I heard most often during my fieldwork, a community-based organization is involved with HIV-related activities not out of a commitment to controlling the epidemic but rather as a means to obtain funding or job security. To accuse a person or an entire organization of eating AIDS rice, then, is to call into question their integrity and belonging in the community of HIV and AIDS workers.

The saying is a play on the socialist-era Chinese idiom "eating from the iron rice bowl" *(tiefanwan)*, which suggested a rice bowl that never went empty and marked a time when the state provided for its citizenry. The transition to a market economy in China inspired many reworkings of this idiom, most notably "eating spring rice" *(qingchunfan)* to describe young women capitalizing on their youth and sex appeal for gainful employment. On one hand, this idiom captured opportunities related to young women's newfound sexual power in a burgeoning market economy; on the other, it reflected shared anxieties around the temporality of these opportunities as "young girls fade into older women" (Hyde 2004, 77; see also Zhang 2000). Similarly, references to an "AIDS rice bowl" communicated opportunities for community-based organizations to grow as a result of the arrival of international HIV donors in the late 1990s and early 2000s and anxieties provoked by their departure and the shift to domestic HIV financing.

The influx of these donors saturated China's HIV sector with abundant resources and funding and directed most of these to community-based organizations. The sudden availability of funding led to a surge in the number of HIV-oriented organizations operating in China's HIV sector.[2] For many community activists and organizational leaders in the sector, the inflow of international HIV support elicited mixed reactions. On one hand, international support marshaled political will and opened up new spaces for advocacy, allowing activists to draw attention, and resources, to those populations enduring the impacts of the HIV epidemic yet which had long been ignored by government officials such as MSM. Furthermore, international donors' preferences for funding community-based organizations legitimized these organizations, repositioning them as key players in the national response to HIV (Kaufman 2009). At the same time, these resources made it possible for hundreds of new groups to be created. Unfortunately, however, these newcomers did not always share the humanitarian ethos to "do good" and "save lives" to which their more established peers subscribed—or at least, this was the belief of many of the more established community leaders at the time of my fieldwork. Many organizers and activists eyed the newer groups and their leaders with distrust, perceiving them to be strictly project based and driven by the availability of funding rather than a real commitment to effecting long-term change in the country.

This distinction between old and new, real and fake, recalled for me a similar contrast made between gay men and money boys as described

by Lisa Rofel (2010), whereby the former condemned the latter for sul-
lying the reputation of Chinese gay men. The gay men claimed that
money boys (in China, *money boys* refers to men who sell sex to other
men) are not gay but rather exploitative and opportunistic, inappro-
priately blurring the boundaries between "sex for money" and "sex for
love," and that their own social standings were tarnished as a result.

Just as members of China's gay community accused money boys
of capitalizing on gayness for monetary gain, so the leaders of China's
longer-established HIV and AIDS organizations accused those who
started after or because of the explosion of international funding of
being in it "for the money." And the phrase "eating AIDS rice" was used
to wage their critique.

Interestingly, Rofel (2010) complicated the "sex for love" versus "sex
for money" binary that informed the understandings of gay men in her
research by proposing another reading of money boys: they "make visible the possibility that this is an economy that produces individuals to
serve the needs of capital accumulation" (453), she claimed, and gay
men may have misrecognized the fact that respectable gay identity has
been as, if not more, embedded in this world of commodified labor and
desire. The metaphorical line between gay men and money boys, Rofel
suggested, was, therefore, slippery. The same slipperiness could be said
to apply to the distinctions drawn between real and fake organizations.
Even as older activists accused newcomers of capitalizing on the epidemic, the former could be said to have benefited as much as, if not
more so than, the latter. Nevertheless, the arrival of so many new organizations in the HIV sector, and especially in relation to serving MSM,
provoked a credibility crisis for all community-based organizations in
China's political landscape.

THE MAKING OF PROJECT-BASED ORGANIZATIONS

Recall that donors like the Global Fund, the Health Fund, and ACF
all invested heavily in community-based organizations to lead the effort in peer-led testing. But they quickly ran into a problem at some
program sites: the absence of community-based organizations serving
MSM. As I discovered in the course of my time spent with the Health
Fund and ACF, in some of the more peripheral, second-tier cities where
they initiated projects, the testing and diagnosis rates among MSM
were consistently low, causing concern among program staff. Because

social pressures for Chinese men to marry and conform to heterosexual norms were amplified in these smaller cities, MSM tended to remain "in hiding" (see chapter 2) among the general public, making them harder to access for health interventions. Given their fears of being exposed or outed, these men were unlikely to seek out HIV services. The solution, at least in some of the Health Fund's program sites, was to work with public health authorities, usually the Chinese CDC, to create or facilitate the creation of locally based organizations that could take up the task of testing—or rather, that could recruit and refer MSM to the Chinese CDC or other VCT sites to get tested for HIV. I had the chance to meet some of the leaders of these newly created organizations during a monitoring trip I took with members of the Health Fund's program team in June 2011. That summer, I traveled with program staff to several sites in southern China. The daily schedule on these trips was generally the same for each site: government meetings in the morning for a briefing on the HIV trends in that city, then a field trip to VCT centers and other community sites where testing takes place, and finally a meeting with community-based organizations to get a sense of their challenges on the ground. On this particular trip, I noticed something that surprised me: none of the MSM groups with which we met existed prior to the arrival of the Health Fund in the region.

The organizations we visited on that trip had, in fact, all been created specifically for the Health Fund's HIV program and primarily to take up the task of recruiting and referring MSM to get tested. In one case, the organization we visited was founded just after the launch of the Health Fund's program in their city. At the time of our meeting in 2011, the Health Fund remained the primary donor to this organization, although staff members told us that they recently applied for, and had been approved for, a Global Fund grant. The director, a young man in his early twenties who was also a college student, had taken on the leadership role a few months prior. Because the organization did not have office space, a local VCT center provided the volunteers with a small room where they could administer pre- and posttest counseling to MSM coming in for HIV tests. The new director served as the only permanent staff, supported by a group of temporary volunteers who assisted with outreach efforts. This outreach involved hosting social events, such as movie nights and karaoke parties, for MSM to promote testing, as well as the use of online tools, such as QQ, to reach MSM.

Sometimes the Chinese CDC would fund the organization's events and administer testing on-site to MSM directly.

The practice of creating project-based organizations is not new in China, nor is it particular to the Health Fund. Timothy Hildebrandt (2011, 983), in his research on the registration process for Chinese social organizations, recounted similar instances of organizations that were created at the behest of the Chinese CDC as a means of "'eating' HIV/AIDS funds," because government institutions were ineligible to access most international HIV resources.[3] Hildebrandt suggested that this practice was more common with organizations serving MSM than with those serving sex workers or people who inject drugs, given that it was for MSM groups that the majority of international funding was earmarked. And yet, it is precisely the "NGO form" as a counterpoint to the state that allows these organizations to operate as flexibly with and apart from the state as they do. Victoria Bernal and Inderpal Grewal (2014) suggest that NGOs are often defined by what they are not, that is, the state, and this characterization tends to obscure their role in actually producing the state. In the case of China, the formation of community-based organizations by government entities but for international donors to carry out tasks for the Chinese CDC exemplifies this "NGO form" insofar as these organizations help produce the state by acting in their interests, and not always in the interests of the community.

I heard similar stories from community leaders about the CDC setting up or creating organizations to "eat AIDS rice." Xu Ping, the director of a health resource center that published an annual directory of NGOs in the sector, described to me how she called organizations to verify their existence as part of the vetting process when putting together the directory. What she found were multiple cases in which, when calling a community-based organization, a CDC staff member answered the phone. "This is how I knew they were fake," she told me. Xu Ping's discoveries resulted in several organizations being removed from the directory each year. From the perspective of long-standing community members like Xu Ping, these newly created groups were driven by economic interests more than by a commitment to HIV prevention and control, given that they were started explicitly to scale up testing among MSM. In her estimation, these project-based organizations contributed little if anything to the wider community beyond technical interventions. Yang Xia, the program officer for the Health Fund, conceded as much, noting that these organizations remained myopic in their missions because they had only ever worked within the context of the Health Fund's program; therefore they understood meeting performance targets for testing MSM but not why MSM should be tested. As an example, Yang Xia pointed to the main activities carried out by local organizations in one city we visited: (1) the hosting of an event where the Chinese CDC administered testing on a fixed day of every month at a local gay bar, (2) the use of QQ and other online tools to recruit men to get tested, and (3) additional social events hosted at different intervention sites across the city. Yang Xia lamented that these activities seemed to be organized around testing only but provided no other forms of support to MSM. To be sure, many of the organizational leaders and staff with whom we met admitted that their events were centered on the Chinese CDC collecting blood samples from MSM and lacked additional counseling or consultations.[4]

The contingent nature of project-based organizations was described especially well by the director of a national tongzhi group who spoke up at a meeting with the Health Fund in 2011: "the problem is that they started out by doing [donors'] work, but they have nothing else to fall back on once these funding sources end. . . . They are organizations chasing after money but without any solid infrastructure to support them." In contrast, the director explained, his organization had an expanded repertoire of services that included managing community health centers and operating online forums, all in support of MSM. "These [project-based] groups do not exist outside of HIV," he concluded, laying bare reliance not just on donors but specifically on testing and, more importantly, collecting performance incentives from MSM. For project-based groups, therefore, MSM bodies circulated as valuable economic commodities.

THE THREAT OF FAKE ORGANIZATIONS

The appearance of project-based organizations emerging out of the Health Fund's MSM testing initiatives sowed distrust among the more established members of the community. More established activists and community leaders decried the project-driven motivations of the newer groups as anathema to the spirit of engaging in community-based work. They criticized these groups for performing "empty" (kong) work, that is, activities that did little to advocate for MSM or control the HIV epidemic. In their estimation, "community" was meant to serve as a space of affective, emotional, and geographic proximity moored in shared values and collective goals (McKay 2018), and community-based organizations needed to reflect those qualities. That project-based groups with unconvincing motives existed and, more importantly, that they garnered HIV resources that could otherwise be used by the longer-established community-based organizations reinforced many activists' and leaders' commitments to policing the boundaries of the MSM community, recognizing some participants and players in China's HIV sector as members and others as outsiders.

Misgivings about project-based organizations were not only related to funding. Critics worried that "fake" groups would undermine the credibility and sustainability of "real" organizations in the wider political landscape, especially as HIV financing increasingly shifted to domestic sources. This latter point is not one to be taken lightly. Community-based organizations have historically been treated with suspicion by the state, although the nature of their relationships with more locally based government agencies like the Chinese CDC vary. Tight, politically enforced control, such as strict registration requirements, restrictions on fund-raising, and geographically and thematically based quotas, were instituted to prevent community-based organizations from participating in "counterrevolutionary" activities, for example (Kaufman 2009, 161). It would follow that any activities perceived to threaten or undermine the standing of community-based organizations would generate controversy, and so they did. These concerns were most clearly articulated by Huang Wei, an activist who was involved with HIV work long before the influx of international donors into China. I first met Huang Wei in 2010 through Jonah, as ACF had been an early donor to his organization. I periodically ran into Huang Wei at different events throughout my time in the field and knew him to be a colorful, somewhat provocative figure who did not shy away from expressing his opinions. He told me that the problem with project-based organizations was that they diverted resources away from "real" groups like his that were dedicated to effecting positive change. He complained that these organizations were just "taking money from them [donors] and not doing any work for it."

By characterizing these groups as not doing "any work," Huang

Wei drew a clear boundary between the groups he felt to be performing meaningful work for the community and others that came into HIV
activities for the money—those that engaged in "empty" work. Like
other leaders of community-based organizations, he blamed international donors for the sudden emergence of project-based groups across
the HIV landscape. For this reason, he welcomed and also pushed for
their departure from China, convinced that "if they leave, at least all
the fake [jia] organizations will disappear and the real [zhen] ones that
are really doing something will stay."

Huang Wei's criticism extended to the Health Fund's program
in particular, which he accused of "ruining civil society" by creating
project-based organizations specifically to test MSM. In his view, performance incentives linked to performance targets stoked competition
and conflict among community-based organizations to test the greatest
number of MSM and identify the greatest number of HIV-positive men
while offering little or nothing else. This strategy, he argued, wasn't
"supporting programs" as part of a wider tool kit of services but rather
turned testing MSM into a tool for making money for organizations.

Huang Wei often spoke to me of "getting [the Health Fund] out of
China," and he went so far as to devise a strategy to do so. He revealed
this plan to me at a chance encounter outside one of ACF's Test, Treat,
and Prevent workshops one weekend in 2011, hoping to enlist my participation (he did not, incidentally). He and other community leaders
planned to draft a letter to the Health Fund requesting a meeting to address their grievances, he told me. "If they refuse," he noted, "then we
will file a complaint directly to their headquarters. Hopefully, that will
get them to respond to us." He expressed confidence that this strategy
would succeed since, as he boasted to me, it was the same one used to
initiate the Global Fund grant freeze (see chapter 3)—an initiative in
which he claimed to have played a key role.

Huang Wei's sentiments resonated across the community of activists and organizers working on HIV- and MSM-related issues. I recall
another moment in a 2011 meeting I attended in Beijing to discuss the
suspension of Global Fund grants and the impact of this suspension on
community-based organizations. At that meeting, a participant bra-
zenly admitted that the organization he represented tested MSM for
money as part of its strategy to survive, given the potential departure of
the Global Fund. His admission elicited swift and strong criticism from

other participants in the room. One man angrily admonished, "This is the problem with the community; people will only do things for money, such as testing; you should do these things because they need to be done, and it shouldn't be tied to money."

It is this same critique that Huang Wei leveraged at ACF's testing projects. He denounced Jonah's acceptance of a grant from the Health Fund, suggesting that taking the grant amounted to ACF abandoning, or at least modifying, its mission as an organization. He lamented, "I used to really like [ACF's] projects," before chiding them for being "just like the Health Fund," insisting that ACF's focus on testing and targets created similar sorts of problems among the community to those engendered by the Health Fund.

These criticisms of MSM testing initiatives underlined an important and yet unexpected outcome of testing interventions: the "instrumentalization" of community-based organizations as technical service delivery agents rather than as stewards of social change (Lai and Spires 2020). For community leaders like Huang Wei, these testing initiatives that appropriated community-based organizations for testing MSM and project-based organizations that performed only testing services were two sides of the same coin insofar as they undermined the capacity of more established groups to effect broader change in China's social and political landscape.

ORIGIN STORIES AS A MARK OF AUTHENTICITY

October 2011: it had been a long day of meetings and filming. By the time Jonah, Zhang Li, and I returned to our hotel, accompanied by Bao Hua and his boyfriend, I was ready to retire for the night. We were traveling in northeastern China to shoot additional footage for a new documentary Jonah was putting together about ACF's Test, Treat, and Prevent project. Because Blue Heart had been an early participant in the project, Jonah asked Bao Hua to arrange a few meetings with some of its beneficiaries, that is, men whom Blue Heart tested and helped get diagnosed over the years as part of ACF's testing project. The men Bao Hua recruited to share their experiences included Xiao Pang, an HIV-positive man whose CD4 count had risen to 160 cells/mm^3 from 20 after he began ART with the support of Blue Heart. Jonah wanted to use the documentary to showcase the lifesaving and life-changing impacts of testing and, more specifically, of peer-led testing among MSM.

Bao Hua invited his boyfriend, Ah Niu, to join us for dinner, because Ah Niu was the original founder of Blue Heart and had given the organization over to Bao Hua to manage, and the two of them later escorted us back to the hotel. Before they could go, however, Jonah, whose energy always exceeded my own, suggested we do a quick debriefing of the day's events, to which we agreed. Assembling in Jonah's hotel room, Bao Hua, Zhang Li, and I casually plopped onto the bed and began to chat informally. The conversation turned to the origins of Blue Heart, and eventually to Bao Hua's personal journey into HIV work by way of his coming into his same-sex desires.

By the time I met Bao Hua and Ah Niu, they were well into their thirties and uninterested in marrying women despite the social pressures for them to do so in their small, second-tier city. Instead, they opted to commit solely to each other. Ah Niu joked that had it not been for his persistence in pursuing Bao Hua, they might not have spent the last ten years together. The two met in a public park back when these venues were hot spots for men seeking other men for casual sex, at a time before the internet and social media were the main tools for arranging sexual encounters. Ah Niu recalled that as he strolled around the park one night, "all of a sudden, I [saw] Bao Hua walking toward me. We looked at each other, and there was a spark of attraction between us. We exchanged a few words, and I invited him back to my place." At Ah Niu's apartment, Bao Hua flung himself onto the bed, signaling his expectations for the encounter. Ah Niu, however, only wanted to talk, so they spent the night conversing instead. The next morning, as Bao Hua prepared to leave, Ah Niu asked him, "When will I see you again?" to which Bao Hua replied nonchalantly, "Next week," code for same time, same place.

The next week, they met at the park, and again, the evening led to conversation but no sex. During the following two months, Ah Niu regularly went to the park in search of Bao Hua, who never showed. Finally, Bao Hua appeared again one night, only to reject Ah Niu's advances, telling him, "There's no sex, so what's the point?" Bao Hua was exclusively interested in one-night stands at the time and saw no reason to pursue anything more with Ah Niu. "He didn't believe that you could fall in love as a tongzhi; he assumed it [same-sex desire] was more of a trend, and that his attraction to men was a phase or something," Ah Niu explained. Yet Ah Niu refused to let Bao Hua go, describing how "I was able to find out where he worked and went directly there to look for him. I was determined to convince Bao Hua to go out with me again." His persistence paid off, and their relationship shaped Bao Hua's acceptance and eventual embrace of his sexuality. "You see," Ah Niu shared, "I had long come to terms with myself as a tongzhi after reading a book that demedicalized homosexuality, stating that it wasn't a disease." He recalled that after reading that book, he became actively involved in advocacy work for MSM, and that activism eventually drew him into HIV work and led him to establish Blue Heart.

Ah Niu emphasized that coming into his sexuality galvanized his activism in a way that had not yet happened for Bao Hua, at least, not at the time of their initial courtship. Bao Hua conceded that it was through their relationship and his gradual acceptance of his same-sex desires that he slowly became immersed in HIV work. He admitted that prior to meeting Ah Niu, he knew nothing of the issues affecting the tongzhi community, a space he entered only after recognizing himself as a man who is attracted to and has sex with other men. Even though it took him years to reconcile these desires, as evidenced by his repeated refusal of Ah Niu's affections and his preference for casual sex only, after Bao Hua learned to accept his same-sex attraction, and once he started to imagine himself as part of a community affected by the epidemic, he quickly became involved in working to address HIV and other health issues, including emotional and psychological care, among MSM, eventually taking over as director of Blue Heart. The process of coming into one's sexual desires acted as a catalyst for Ah Niu's activism and, as it turned out, for Bao Hua's too.

Bao Hua's story mirrors those of other community leaders I met who became activists at a time when same-sex relations were medically pathologized and politically risky and the HIV epidemic itself was largely ignored by the Chinese government. I once heard an activist say, "We did this work back when there were no projects available," stressing early activists' drive to do something when there were no political or economic resources to be had. Rather, they did this work because "there was a need," as another community leader expressed. Indeed, the earliest HIV-related organizations emerged in the 1990s, long before international donors arrived, and certainly prior to any political attention being given to the HIV epidemic, much less to MSM.

* * * * *

Origin stories located groups like Blue Heart in the tongzhi community long before the introduction of global health categories like "MSM" came onto the scene and prior to the arrival of global health donors that targeted MSM for HIV interventions. Early organizations in China's HIV sector emerged organically out of a social collective formed by sexual and affective ties that inspired activists' commitments to "doing good" because there was a need, and not because there was funding. Community activists at the time of my fieldwork often invoked this temporal past and their participation in it as a way to validate the authenticity or "realness" of the organizations for which they worked and volunteered. I once heard the director of an NGO admonish the staff of a newly formed group for asking for additional resources: "In the beginning, our group didn't have much funding, and we relied on volunteers. It was only recently that we started to generate any funding, but we started out doing tongzhi projects because we felt there was a need, and we did it without any funding at all."

"MSM," as a relatively new moniker in China and a global health category that did not differentiate sexual alterities, came to stand, at least among the more established community members, as a marker for an organization's (in)authenticity. Blue Heart, for example, considered itself to be an LGBT group that provided emotional and other health-related services to its community, including but not limited to testing and other interventions. Even though its primary demographic remained MSM, the organization situated itself as part of a wider collective effort to advocate for the rights of sexual minorities in the country. I became starkly aware of the distinction between organizations that targeted MSM and those that served tongzhi during a conversation I had with a community activist, when I mistakenly referred to his NGO as an MSM one. He corrected me abruptly, clarifying that his NGO was a "tongzhi group and always has been." He explained his organization's participation in testing projects (including ACF and the Health Fund) as one part of what it did, making it clear that its priorities extended beyond the technical aspect of administering testing, instead integrating testing into a greater repertoire of services for tongzhi.

For many activists, staff, and volunteers involved in China's fight to reduce HIV transmission among MSM, origin stories served an important purpose. They served as a referendum on authenticity, marking as "real" those organizations that emerged from lived experiences and personal connections to communities. The personal journeys of people like Bao Hua ensured, to some degree, that these organizations would continue their work long after the funding and other resources for that work had faded. In contrast, the precarious positionalities of project-based organizations suggested that they would exist only as long as their funding lasted and that such organizations would be unable to create long-term change. It was for this reason that community leaders were especially aggrieved when project-based groups received funding from international donors. They were taking, it seemed, from "real" organizations able to advance greater goals. In distinguishing the authentic and the long term from the inauthentic and the short term, origin stories also performed important boundary work, reinscribing belonging as accessible to certain kinds of individuals and organizations while inaccessible to others.

COMMUNITY AND THE POLITICS OF PLACE:
YOU DON'T BELONG HERE

The origin stories that adjudicated belonging for groups like Blue Heart had the opposite effect for ACF, and for Jonah in particular. For as long as I have known him, Jonah has always been strongly committed to empowering communities to care for, support, and advocate for themselves by working to give the members of these communities the skills and tools needed to do so. I gradually came to understand how his personal journey as a gay Asian American man living through the HIV epidemic in the United States had shaped the values that guided ACF's work. Take, for example, ziworentong, the self-affirmation project I described in chapter 2. Jonah recounted that this project transpired out of his experiences with gay support groups in the United States, groups that instantiated the very idea of community. Inspired by these models, he drew on his former experiences to design the kinds of interventions he believed to be the most effective in addressing not only the public health but also the social needs of MSM in China.

Jonah has long viewed himself to be a part of the community of activists advocating for the rights of MSM in China and fighting to address the impacts of HIV on these men. Indeed, all of ACF's projects and resources and most of Jonah's labor are invested in China, even though he spends only half of his time in the country. Despite this geo-graphic distance, Jonah, like many other activists working in the HIV sector, is motivated by a humanitarian ethic to save lives, especially as a gay man who lost his partner and many friends to AIDS. Jonah once said about the epidemic, "even if you were not involved in it, you were still involved in it," underscoring the depth to which HIV affected gay men's social worlds. To him, the very idea of "community" is one that transcends geographic borders and instead is anchored in the "spirit," as he called it, to do something.

This spirit engendered the genesis of ACF. After his partner passed, Jonah became involved with various social groups formed for gay Asian American men in the United States, many of whom traced their lin-eage back to China, although most had been raised in the United States and knew little of China. What began as a social gathering for men to talk about topics that affected their daily lives changed after one of the members came across a news story exposing the blood scandals in cen-tral China, through which thousands of rural farmers contracted HIV after donating (in return for remuneration) blood and plasma to com-mercial collection stations. Galvanized by a sense of belonging to an "imagined community" (Anderson 1983) based on Chinese heritage, and which transgressed national borders, this story motivated several of the men at the gathering to do something. Over time, the social col-lective transitioned into a smaller group of core members motivated to provide aid in response to the HIV epidemic in China. Thus ACF was born.

It is no coincidence that the origins of ACF, emerging out of a small community of gay Asian American men, shaped the strong community-oriented focus of the organization, especially under Jonah's leader-ship. Jonah explained that the founding members knew from the start that "we wanted innovation; we wanted social change," and that goal manifested in the decision to support community-based organizations that could create relief efforts for HIV-impacted communities. Recall that ACF's Test, Treat, and Prevent project originated from a desire for peer-led testing as an alternative to clinical testing at public health institutions, where men typically experienced discrimination. By en-abling community-based testing, men would be able to take control of their health and gain a sense of belonging to a community of others "just like them." It was this kind of innovative and community-oriented thinking, Jonah said, that attracted the Health Fund to their project and resulted in a generous grant to support the initiative.

ACF's acceptance of the Health Fund grant generated heated controversy among community activists. To some, like Huang Wei, ACF's project mirrored too closely the Health Fund's emphasis on technical services and achieving numbers, even though ACF's testing project asked grantees to report numbers, not meet targets; Huang Wei argued that the funding should go directly to community-based organizations rather than an entity like ACF, which, in many ways, could be considered a donor itself given its financial support to other organizations. Jonah dismissed these criticisms and explained that most of the funding went directly to community-based organizations. Another criticism, that of Fu Xiao (introduced earlier) and other activists who shared his thinking, was that ACF's projects were too "feelings based" and should focus more intensely on providing technical, health-related information about how to prevent HIV transmission. And still to others, such as the HIV resource center director Xu Ping (introduced earlier), ACF was undeserving of funding not because of its activities but because of geography: ACF was a U.S.-based organization.

I had heard about Xu Ping long before I met her. A community activist I knew well once referred to her as part of the "gang of four," a play on the political faction that rose to power and terror during the Chinese cultural revolution. This "gang" counted among its members Xu Ping, Huang Wei, and Fu Xiao. According to Jonah, the group commanded a lion's share of HIV resources, power, and influence in China's HIV activism community. Xu Ping's NGO, for example, once served as the only platform to disseminate election information for the Global Fund's country-coordinating mechanism, the governing body for its grants, a role that invited controversy amid accusations that the organization monopolized the flow of information (Galler 2015). Over the years, however, Xu Ping's NGO downsized, due in part to the decline in HIV resources that had affected most groups in the country. By the time I met Xu Ping, she was the only full-time staff member of that organization.

Xu Ping's discontent, Jonah told me, centered on the Health Fund's grant to ACF. It seemed Xu Ping took issue with the grant because, as she told Jonah, he did not belong "in the community" (*bushi shequ*) and therefore should not be accepting, or rather did not have a right to accept, HIV resources from donors in the country. I misunderstood her comments to mean that Jonah should not be entitled to take resources targeting MSM, so I pointed out that he himself was gay and ACF's projects supported these men. "How is that not in the community?" I asked. However, Jonah clarified that her issue was not with his sexuality or ACF's projects but rather had to do with his nationality and part-time residency. In other words, ACF, and, by extension, Jonah, was based in the United States, not in China, making ACF a foreign organization and not "of here." I reiterated that all of ACF's projects and resources were invested in China and Chinese MSM. "Yes," Jonah agreed, "but Xu Ping considers herself more *in the community* than me because her NGO is located in China."

Xu Ping's concern for Jonah's geographic positionality reinscribed national borders as a key criterion for belonging "in the community" and mediating one's right to access HIV resources within China—even if those resources originated from outside of the country. Her designation of ACF as foreign recalled, for me, the origin stories about HIV in the 1980s and 1990s, linking the virus to "exotic" places like Africa and Haiti (see Farmer 1992; Sontag 1989; Treichler 1999) and which were used politically to fortify geographic borders. Xu Ping utilized similar narratives to characterize ACF as undeserving of grants in China, reinforcing nationalism by casting ACF as an outsider—as not Chinese and not of here. In so doing, Xu Ping rejected ACF from her own imagined community, one buttressed by geographic and national proximity. She argued that funding was given to ACF at the expense of more deserving, domestic organizations in the country, for example, her NGO. In effect, she accused ACF of unethically consuming from the AIDS rice bowl, diverting resources away from "local" groups that were unlikely to have access to the "global" network of donors available to ACF. As Xu Ping told Jonah, "donor funding in China is meant for Chinese organizations, not foreign ones." Jonah admitted that he heard this critique from other community activists as well.

Xu Ping's exclusion of ACF and Jonah indexed deeper anxieties about the present and future of organizations like her own in a shifting public health landscape that increasingly favored technical and performance-based interventions, including HIV testing. As a resource center that positioned itself as an advocacy platform, Xu Ping's NGO had all but been cut out of international support, and the organization was equally ill positioned to receive domestic funding as the Chinese CDC turned more and more to community-based organizations for service delivery.

Jonah challenged the criterion by which Xu Ping defined (and excluded him from) community, asserting that belonging was not bound by place or geography but rather was anchored in a "spirit," something that approximated a moral calling. "I consider myself to be more in the community than [she is]," he stated, "not because I am gay but because I understand the needs of the community." He pointed to ACF's Test, Treat, and Prevent project as embodying that kind of spirit because it not only addressed the needs of MSM but also contributed to greater goals that advanced the standing of community-based organizations in China. Here he drew on the narrative of "community" promoted by activists like Huang Wei, community as driven by a greater mission and collective goals and not just testing or other technical interventions.

Jonah explained the scaling back of Xu Ping's NGO as the result of her lack of community spirit. He described how she recently fired almost all of her staff and had become increasingly "possessive" of her projects, wary that other people might steal her ideas to attain funding. "All of the funding for her NGO goes to her, not the organization," he alleged, casting doubt on the community-driven mission of her NGO and suggested instead that her personal gain rendered the NGO project based. He criticized her suspicions as "going against the spirit of this kind of work," noting that "you should not be trying to keep projects to yourself; if they are good, you should want to spread them around so more people can benefit from them." Jonah juxtaposed his desire to expand ACF's projects to Xu Ping's impulse to guard her projects and, he implied, her funding.

Xu Ping, on the other hand, offered a different account of her circumstances. In her version, she recounted how she had been brought into the NGO years earlier to revive it, as it had been in dismal financial straits at the time she assumed the director role. A key donor had just departed, and because most staff salaries had been paid from that source, this put a significant strain on the organization's operations. Consequently, Xu Ping was forced to lay off many staff members and transition others to part-time positions to keep the organization afloat. Existing funding streams at the time came primarily from domestic sources, although Xu Ping expressed a desire to diversify and gain support from international donors, a desire that may have contributed to her displeasure at ACF's grant success. Her personal income, she revealed, did not come from the NGO but rather from independent consultancy work she undertook. It was, perhaps, for this reason that she became concerned that "people steal ideas," as she told me, before asking me not to share her project ideas out of fear they might get funded elsewhere.

In Xu Ping's understanding, Jonah, whom she criticized for "not being here all the time," did not share the collective history that moored Xu Ping and other Chinese activists and organizers working in China's HIV sector to a singular community. "I have been working in this field for years," she told me, recalling the sentiments of those other community activists who began their work at a time when political will was wanting and economic resources were few. Her observations recalled for me Donald Moore's (1998) descriptions of land rights struggles in Zimbabwe in the late 1990s. In his writings, Moore told the story of Angela, who denied the legitimacy of the chief to rule by reasoning that he lived outside of the territories under colonial eviction during a critical moment in Zimbabwe's history and did not participate in the struggles to maintain the community's land rights. For Angela, as for Xu Ping, belonging was situated in and circumscribed by shared, emplaced historical experience. Jonah, based partly in the United States, could not and did not experience the struggle that many community-based organizations went through in their fight against HIV as it was lived by those based full time in China—at least, according to Xu Ping—and this made him undeserving.

In contrast, Jonah's counterconstruction of community embeds his belonging by virtue of spirit, that is, the spirit of a collective of activists and organizations fighting against HIV and for MSM in China.

Toward the end of my fieldwork, I ran into Xu Ping at the Health Fund, just as I headed out to lunch. After briefly chatting in the hallway, before she turned into a meeting room, she said to me, "I just sent you a message. Did you get it?" I replied that I had not yet checked my text messages and had left my phone at my desk, and I asked what it was about. She smiled mysteriously and said, "Just check your messages." After I returned from lunch, I picked up my phone and indeed found a message from Xu Ping. It read, "Good news! The project we discussed today is getting funded by the Health Fund."

CONCLUSION

This chapter has examined the aftermath of MSM testing as it unraveled among the community of MSM targeted by this intervention.
Community-based organizations in China dedicated to reducing HIV
transmission among MSM burgeoned over the years as international
donors arrived and brought with them an abundance of HIV-related
funding. This funding provided these organizations with increased
legitimacy and a greater sense of belonging in the national political
sphere, and international donors' support has been particularly beneficial to MSM groups, expanding their ability to advocate for their communities; as one activist admitted to me, "HIV gave tongzhi a chance to
demand human rights." However, these international donors and their
preferences for technical interventions (i.e., HIV testing) and countable returns also led to a splintering of the community. Activists and
organizers who had worked with few resources and little to no recognition before the arrival of international donors blamed the donors for
a rise in newly formed *project*-based organizations, which they distinguished from more established *community*-based organizations. That is,
project-based organizations were characterized as those that "eat AIDS
rice" or were in it for the money—organizations that were perceived to
take funding away from groups and treated MSM bodies as economic
commodities. These project-based organizations were more singularly
focused on testing MSM and collecting performance incentives set by
international donors and the Chinese CDC and rarely on providing additional services outside of testing parameters. Testing, although important to controlling the epidemic, was often carried out in isolation
from other health-related services and did not always address other
issues driving HIV transmission among MSM. These project-based
organizations, at least from the standpoint of established community
leaders, threatened to undercut the abilities of community-based organizations to engage in advocacy-oriented work, instead reducing these
groups to technical service providers.

The tensions described in this chapter evoked a deeper politics of
belonging that reinforced and reinscribed boundaries for membership.
Established activists who have long sought to make legitimate their
community as made up of individuals driven by humanitarian ethos
rather than funding perceived project-based organizations with suspi-

cion, wary that the latter may undermine their credibility as mission directed and community oriented. Naisargi Dave (2012, 60) has argued that this process of rendering communities "authentic and representable" has become even more prioritized as these communities accumulate social, and, in this instance, political, value. As I have described in this chapter, global health interventions do not always unfold in expected ways. In the next chapter, I trace what happens after some MSM are tested, and test positive, for HIV.

FIVE

LIVING WITH HIV
AS MSM IN CHINA

THE PUSH TO SCALE UP TESTING among MSM not only placed these men at the center of health interventions; it also brought to the fore questions of sexual practice among MSM. The struggles of the men described in this chapter illustrate how they sought to reconcile their social obligations as Chinese men and their same-sex desires as MSM in the aftermath of an HIV-positive diagnosis. The decisions they made reflect the complexities and contradictions of their everyday practices that aim to conjoin caring for the self with caring for others. For these men, their decisions moved beyond safe sexual practices but were articulated around how they felt they ought to live as HIV-positive MSM. Should they live openly as same-sex-desiring men with other men, or should they remain in their heteronormative lifestyles as socially obligated of them? Do they inform their spouses or their families of their HIV status, or do they remain silent so as to protect those they care for from public shame? Their stories are not just about doing the "right thing" but reflect deeper struggles with how to live within their social worlds. This chapter therefore asks, what does it mean to live as an HIV-positive Chinese MSM?

The answer to this question arises from the nexus of two forces: the scaling up of testing that targeted MSM and the social expectations for Chinese men to carry on their lineage in society. Historically in China, personhood is realized within a context characterized by family and social relations rather than as a discrete, autonomous self, as in many Euro-American contexts (Chou 2001). This construction of personhood has been especially pronounced for Chinese men, given that establishing a heteronormative family is a defining characteristic of Chinese masculinity.

Market reforms in the 1970s catalyzed a sexual revolution that altered traditional notions of such personhood and freed, if only somewhat, individuals to pursue their personal, and sexual, interests. For MSM, the effects have been tempered by still-rigid heterosexual norms and notions of masculinity. Moreover, HIV and AIDS added to this constraint since interventions to control the spread of HIV increasingly placed MSM bodies and their same-sex sexual practices at the forefront. As public health discourse further medicalized same-sex sexual behaviors and men came to inhabit "MSM" as a global health category and an emerging selfhood, MSM's making of themselves "into a certain kind of person" (Laidlaw 2002, 322) became ever more meaningful. Just as scaling up HIV testing of MSM transformed men's bodies into commodities of care, the rise of testing interventions also animated MSM's transformation into proper, "morally recognizable subjects" (Dave 2012, 6). The form that recognition took, however, varied.

I take as my focal point the experiences of MSM after they get tested, and after they receive an HIV-positive diagnosis. I particularly attend to their struggles to respond accordingly, for themselves and for others. Many of these men were tested as part of wider testing initiatives described in the earlier chapters. I foreground their struggles because theirs are the stories not reflected in the metrics collected by community-based organizations. While numbers can tell stories about people, numbers can also obscure stories about people. These are stories that enable us to see beyond the numbers: like how health interventions, including testing MSM, unravel in the lives of men targeted by its implementation. Stories also best illustrate how deeply entwined the lives and the decisions of MSM are with the shifting social and cultural norms and values that shape their daily lives. These stories underscore how testing alone is insufficient to prevent HIV.

I examine in this chapter the different ways in which MSM understand and respond to an HIV-positive diagnosis in their everyday lives. I locate these practices in moments of self-reflection regarding men's same-sex desires, in actions taken to fulfill their social obligations as Chinese men, and in silences about their HIV status as they pursue what they consider to be "proper" lives. I suggest that MSM's endeavors are tied to and inflected by "MSM" as a global health category and emerging selfhood. This chapter builds on the previous chapter, in which I explored the aftereffects of MSM testing and its impacts across the community of organizers, activists, staff, volunteers, and others who were tasked with promoting and performing HIV tests on the ground. I now attend to how MSM, specifically HIV-positive men, as the recipients of testing implemented by community-based organizations, enact similar modalities of inclusion and exclusion in their everyday lives. I came to understand the decisions made (at the time) by the men with whom I worked as a way to articulate social and cultural belonging according to the norms of Chinese society. I am reminded of a self-identified tongzhi I met in spring 2011 who, after discovering he was HIV-positive, admitted to still planning to get married and start a family, and yet wrestled with whether to inform his future wife of his HIV status, reflecting "probably not, [as] this isn't something easy to tell." This man, as with many of the men I describe in this book, asked himself, what kind of life should I live as an HIV-positive Chinese MSM?

SEX AND THE AMBIVALENT CHINESE SUBJECT

It is not an understatement to say that the economic growth and transformation of China since the market reforms in the 1970s reverberated across all aspects of daily life for Chinese citizens. These reforms not only dismantled the "iron rice bowl" once safeguarded by state-owned enterprises; they also catalyzed profound shifts in Chinese subjectivities and notions of personhood. The answer to the question "who am I?" once circumscribed by a set of social relations centered on family and kin and later tied to a collectivist and socialist state gave way to notions of an enterprising self, at once self-governing and self-reliant. This change gave rise to a deeper "quest for meaning in everyday life," as Arthur Kleinman (2010, 1075) described, and created new interest in remaking the self, amid a fluid and fluctuating moral landscape within which personhood is shaped.

Yan Yunxiang (2011) examined the shifting moral landscape in China following the reforms of the 1970s to describe how a once collective morality characterized by responsibility was being replaced by an individual morality that incorporated personal interests, individual rights, and self-development as good and worthy. New and growing individual desires collided with yearnings for a collective morality of the past. For instance, Yan showed how individuals involved with food safety scandals or the production of fake and faulty goods in China justified their actions as part of the pursuit of individual success, ostensibly indifferent to the consequences to others as a result of their actions. But rather than juxtaposing collective against individual morality, Yan's analysis illustrated how personal interests are sedimented into existing ethical regimes that remain, still today, deeply ingrained in Chinese lives. He underlined how living a moral and ethical life became all the more ambiguous for Chinese citizens.

This ambiguity is especially pronounced in the domain of sexuality. The economic reforms of the 1970s had an important effect not only on remaking personhood but also on how citizens conceived of their personal sexual pleasures. The opening up of the country gave individuals license, so to speak, to pursue their financial interests and act on their sexual desires simultaneously. Some scholars have characterized this freedom as a "sexual revolution" (Pan 2006; Zhang 2011).[1] The seeking out of sexual pleasure was no longer seen to be an obstacle to success but rather became a means to it. Take for instance practices of *yingchou* whereby entertaining and soliciting sex workers became an integral part of conducting business with government officials. Elanah Uretsky (2016) argued that *yingchou,* rather than practiced out of sexual desire, served as a way to mark loyalties to the state within a new economic system that distributed rewards based on market logics. In postsocialist China, arguably, financial and sexual pursuits increasingly went hand in hand.

To be sure, sex became increasingly visible and available, especially to those willing to pay, as new spaces for sexual consumption (pornography, sexually oriented media and literature, sex shops, dating sites) proliferated across the country (Ho 2010; Jeffreys 2006). It could be said that a new ethos took hold, one that celebrated, rather than repressed, the pursuit of sexual pleasure. Everett Zhang (2011) pointed to the many types of premarital and extramarital arrangements that have multiplied in postsocialist China, including sex work, keeping mistresses, and other forms of sexual relationships that extend beyond traditional heterosexual, monogamous marriage and allow individuals to pursue a widening range of sexual interests. And yet, this new sexual ethos limited these freedoms to a select few. The sexual revolution resulted in a kind of tolerance for, though by no means a social acceptance of, same-sex relations, for example. By the 1990s, China saw a rising cohort of men and woman taking on gay and lesbian identities

(Rofel 1999). In time, gay-friendly spaces started to appear, and some public attitudes slowly began to shift. These advancements should not be mistaken to mean that same-sex relations achieved acceptance, so much as they were part of a wider landscape of sexual consumption made possible by market reforms. As Li Yinhe (2006) demonstrated, the social risks of exposing men's same-sex sexual activities operated as a far more effective tool to regulate same-sex relations than any legal ramifications could have done; the continued stigmatization and hiddenness of same-sex relations even after the so-called sexual revolution speaks to the entrenchment of those "social risks."

Foucault argued that freedom is always of a "definite, historically produced kind" insofar as it is modeled after practices found in and reinforced by culture and society (Laidlaw 2002, 323). For Chinese MSM, this freedom has been mediated in two ways. First has been by testing interventions that reproduced cultural narratives of MSM as immoral and sexually promiscuous, thereby demanding a (self-)disciplining of their same-sex sexual practices. This (self-)policing of MSM's sexual practices potentially meant, second, that MSM had to take up their social roles as Chinese men who were filial sons, husbands, and fathers despite their sexual preferences.

MSM frequently seek out heterosexual relationships that permit, or at least provide cover for, them to pursue their same-sex desires. By doing so, these men reflect the newly formed "desiring subject" (Rofel 2007) who goes after, but also bears responsibility for, their personal choices—that is, choices that are consistently tempered by state ideologies that continue to inform what should and should not be desired, even as the state retreats from directly intervening in the private lives of citizens (Li and Ong 2008). I suggest that the desires and decisions of the men with whom I worked were underpinned by these competing ideologies.

SELF-DISCIPLINE AND THE RIGHT TO SEX FOR HIV-POSITIVE MSM

The sexual revolution I described led to two critical breaks in the sexual lives of Chinese citizens. First came the uncoupling of sex from reproduction, enabling individuals to seek out sexual pleasure as an end to itself. In effect, sex no longer had to be confined to the institution of marriage or carried out for the purposes of reproduction but could now be pursued for the sake of pleasure. The second break separated sex from love, thus allowing individuals to reimagine the value of sex in their lives. Pan Suiming (2006) pointed to two historical moments that led to these transformations: the one-child policy that actively restricted reproduction (though not sex) among couples, making it possible to envision sex for pleasure, and the Marriage Law of 1980, which allowed for divorce on the grounds of loss of love or affection, freeing individuals to engage in sex for the sake of sex.

These changes marked an important step in validating, at least for heterosexual individuals, the pursuit of sexual pleasures, pushing the boundaries of acceptable mores. For MSM, however, these societal shifts had contradictory effects, allowing, on one hand, for more opportunities for same-sex sexual consumption, yet, on the other hand, provoking ambivalence around proper and improper sexual conduct. The latter generally manifested as internalized homophobia and elicited "self-criticism" among many of these men (Zheng 2015), who sought to distance themselves from the perceived promiscuity of MSM by idealizing monogamous, heterosexual relationships as an alternative to meeting their companionship needs (Kong 2011; Sun, Farrer, and Choi 2006). For some of these men, the increasing rates of HIV in their community only reinforced their presumptions about MSM and underlined the need to (self-)police sexual practices.

Take, for instance, the comments made by a young man on a panel I attended during the 2014 Shanghai Pride. The event was one of the longest-running LGBTQ festivals in China, intended to celebrate and legitimize same-sex relations.[2] This man, a doctoral student at a nearby university who publicly identified as "gay" (in English), denounced the "right now attitude" toward sex exhibited by men in his community. He argued that condoms are ineffective against HIV if men do not use them and alleged that men in his community did not use them. To this point, he criticized that "the men in our circle [quanzi] are more interested in instant gratification," blaming this attitude for the increasing rates of HIV among MSM.

I came across similar sentiments throughout my research. A common grievance I heard came from leaders of MSM-oriented community-based organizations, who complained about the libertine sexual activities of their staff and volunteers, especially with men coming into the organization to seek out testing services. One director criticized his staff and volunteers for engaging in casual sexual encounters after hours on the premises; he found their conduct not only unprofessional but morally distasteful. In another instance, participants attending an ACF workshop chided other men for treating the event as an opportunity to "sleep around with each other," as they put it. The many denouncements beget the question, how should MSM act, especially as their bodies come to signify both the spread and containment of the HIV epidemic? The young man on the panel left me reflecting upon two points at once. First was the implication that there is a need to police MSM's sexual practices but not desires; by assailing men's promiscuity and unsafe sexual practices, the young man delineated the boundaries of proper and improper conduct for MSM. Second, his criticisms rendered sexual pleasure as a thing to be acted upon only under certain conditions (not "right now," for example).

These tensions around MSM's sexual practices were especially pronounced for HIV-positive MSM, and studies show that these men are often held more accountable than heterosexuals for their infections (Neilands, Steward, and Choi 2008). I recall a particularly jarring moment for me during fieldwork when, over lunch with a friend, the topic of my research came up and she immediately remarked, "If these men get AIDS, then they deserve it." Her words shocked me; this friend had, after all, helped me organize HIV workshops in the past and had expressed compassion for the discrimination experienced by people living with HIV. I expressed my surprise at her comments, and she clarified, "If you contract HIV through blood transfusion, then it's not your fault. But these men go out and have unprotected sex and get infected; then they deserve to get AIDS." Her compassion, I realized, was reserved only for a privileged minority of people publicly designated to be "innocent" in contracting HIV. But it also reproduced the cultural narrative that only certain kinds of people contract HIV in the first place. Her comments reflected a sentiment that prevailed among the general public in China, including some MSM. As Feng, Wu, and Detels (2010) found in their study, a common presumption among these men is that those who test positive must be self-indulgent and sexually licentious, that is, they must have multiple sexual partners.

For men like Xiao Lin, these particular narratives about MSM informed his advocacy for sexual self-discipline, a commitment he made in the aftermath of an HIV-positive diagnosis in 2009. Xiao Lin, a self-identified tongzhi in his twenties (introduced in chapter 2), admitted to knowing little about HIV or his risk as an MSM until he came into contact with testing campaigns organized by community-based organizations in his city. After testing HIV-positive, he joined a support group for people living with HIV started by one of ACF's grantees, which is where I first met him in October 2011. That day, Jonah, Zhang Li, and I met with four members of the support group to which Xiao Lin belonged to hear about their experiences living with HIV. Xiao Lin rushed into the room nearly thirty minutes into the conversation, breathless and apologetic for being late. He explained that he had been next door waiting to pick up his medications at the infectious disease hospital located only yards away from where we were sitting, after a brief stay there due to some HIV complications.

Jonah calmly reassured Xiao Lin that we had only just started and invited Xiao Lin to join us in the small circle of chairs we had arranged in the middle of the single-room concrete building. Jonah explained that the men were sharing how they contracted HIV and asked Xiao Lin, "Do you know how you contracted HIV?" Xiao Lin nodded and shared with the group: "I contracted HIV from my former bf [boyfriend]. I found out I was HIV-positive about two years ago. We had been together for about five years, but we split up briefly because he was having problems with his family and moved away, so we separated. Later, he returned, and we got back together. But during the time we were apart, he had unprotected sex with other men, and then transmitted HIV to me when we reconciled." He then paused for a moment, as if reflecting, and then continued: "After I learned I was HIV-positive, I stopped having sex altogether. I don't believe in sleeping around." He pointed out that "there are only two ways to prevent HIV: using condoms and being in a long-term relationship. But I no longer have sex anymore."

Xiao Lin's admission both surprised and confused Jonah, who gently pushed back. "I disagree with you," he stated, pointing out how "you said yourself that you contracted HIV from a long-term boyfriend; how did that [relationship] protect you against HIV?" though Jonah noted that there was little Xiao Lin could have done in that circumstance. Instead, he insisted that Xiao Lin could and should still enjoy sex, precisely because he knew his HIV status and therefore could safely engage in sex to prevent transmitting HIV to another person. Getting tested and practicing safe sex, according to Jonah, made it possible for Xiao Lin, as an HIV-positive man, to engage in sexual activity responsibly by not knowingly transmitting the virus to another person. In his rationale, Jonah drew a careful distinction between what he perceived to be the morality of a long-term relationship and the ethics of practicing safe sex as a part of one's everyday life.

Xiao Lin nevertheless defended his stance, contending that "I don't think having random sex and using condoms is good," laying emphasis on the (im)morality of casual sexual encounters with or without a condom. For him, the issue was not the use of condoms so much as the act of sex itself under certain conditions. Xiao Lin's distrust of condoms as an effective barrier outside of a long-term relationship mirrors findings by other scholars regarding condom use and understandings of condoms among Chinese MSM. For many men, the use of condoms signaled potential seropositivity or the presence of another STI of a sexual partner; this presumption holds especially true for men in long-term relationships. For a man to insist upon condom use in a monogamous relationship implied, to many, infidelity, or at least cast doubt upon a partner's fidelity. The absence of condom use, in contrast, symbolized to many monogamous couples mutual trust in each other, giving men the perception that they and their partners were at low risk for contracting HIV (Choi et al. 2004; Zhou 2006; see also Ma et al. 2013). It is worth remembering that Xiao Lin's partner engaged in unprotected sex during their separation, and presumably not during their partnership.

Xiao Lin and Jonah's debate drew into sharp relief the right to sexual pleasure for MSM, in particular, for HIV-positive men. I read this disagreement as indexing a deeper issue, that is, the question of appropriate sexual conduct for HIV-positive MSM. Xiao Lin's decision to pursue abstinence after his diagnosis signaled to me an intentional practice to make himself into a proper MSM who does not "sleep around," to use his words, and is committed to long-term relationships.[3] This choice was underpinned by the cultural narratives that portrayed MSM as sexually promiscuous and risky. It could be said that Xiao Lin is not unlike other MSM who idealize monogamous, heterosexual relationships, not as a manifestation of internalized homophobia in his case but perhaps as the only other model available to him. His practice of abstinence can be understood as a technology of the self (Foucault 1988), an active self-fashioning undertaken to make himself into a certain kind of person. By outlining the conditions under which he felt sex to be acceptable, he signaled his belonging as a responsible sexual citizen.

TESTING AND THE PURSUIT OF SEXUAL PLEASURE AMONG MSM

The debate described herein did not get resolved, as Jonah and Xiao Lin never did come to an agreement. But their debate revealed the many possibilities, ambivalences, and contradictions that arose when MSM sought to reconcile "proper" sexual conduct in light of an HIV-positive diagnosis. Jonah remained a steadfast believer in the right of MSM to pursue and enjoy sex, regardless of their HIV status or their same-sex sexual practices; as he often said to me, "I don't care if men have multiple or short-term [sexual] partners; I only care if they know their HIV status, so they can have sex safely." The right to sex, according to Jonah, was enabled by HIV testing, as testing provided men with knowledge that allowed them to pursue sexual exploits safely and responsibly.

For Jonah, testing was always a tool of empowerment and a technology of the self insofar as it permitted "individuals to effect by their own means or with the help of others a certain number of operations on their own bodies and souls, thoughts, conduct, and way of being, so as to transform themselves in order to attain a certain state of happiness, purity, wisdom, perfection, or immortality" (Foucault 1988, 18). Technologies can take on different forms, but they are practiced in pursuit of an ethical project to remake oneself into a certain kind of person (Foucault 1986; see also Laidlaw 2002). In this regard, testing among MSM elicited knowledge about one's HIV status as part of one's self as an MSM, that in turn prompted men to modulate their conduct, as it did for Xiao Lin.

It is this principle that informed most of ACF's projects, from Test, Treat, and Prevent to ziworentong (self-affirmation). Testing, at least for Jonah, was more than the extension of a technical intervention into a population to reduce HIV transmission; it was a technology that became deeply entwined with and shaped by MSM's conceptions of the self. This relationship is perhaps best illustrated by two personal stories that Jonah shared with me during my time in the field. Recall that in November 2011, I attended a ziworentong workshop that ACF organized for its grantees. As described in chapter 2, at that particular meeting, men shared their best and worst sexual experiences as a way to help them identify and renounce those sexual practices that put men at risk for contracting HIV. In that meeting, Jonah shared a story about one of his worst sexual experiences:

> I was on vacation in Europe, and while there, I visited a local bath-house one night. Inside, I met this man who was nothing short of Adonis. He was beautiful, he had rock solid abs. . . . He led me into a sort of back room, and then we proceeded to have sex. Afterwards, he just got up and left, without anything more intimate. The whole experience felt so impersonal; I felt like I had been used. That was one of the worst sexual experiences of my life.

In contrast, he then described one of the best sexual experiences he ever had:

> With my partner, who passed away from AIDS. It was when he had already become very sick; he was no longer able to have sex with me because of all the medications he was taking. One night, when we were in bed together, my partner leaned over and gave me a hand job. Afterwards, as we lay next to each other talking, he told me that he knew I had sexual needs, and even though he could no longer have [penetrative] sex with me, this was the very least he could do for me. I was so moved. It was one of my best moments because even at his weakest, my partner was still thinking of me.

Jonah juxtaposed these two distinct moments to then emphasize the salience of testing and, more importantly, of knowing, in the pursuit of sexual pleasure. After sharing his stories, he described the shame he felt following his momentary encounter in the European bathhouse, shame laced by his awareness that he had failed to care for himself and put himself and his sexual partner at risk for HIV. He confessed to the group that the encounter entailed no sharing of personal details, including their respective HIV or other STI statuses, and no use of condoms. Instead, the encounter served merely as a sexual transaction cloaked in anonymity—precisely the kind of anonymity that drives HIV-risky behaviors among MSM (Altman et al. 2012; Beyrer et al. 2011). Jonah's remorse, he again conceded, came not from the sexual encounter itself but from not knowing his HIV status and engaging in unprotected sex.

His second story served as a corrective to the first one by under-scoring that testing was a tool that allowed him to seek sexual pleasure in a safe and responsible manner. As he told the story, Jonah detailed the intimacy cultivated between him and his partner, an intimacy facilitated by knowing their respective HIV statuses and seeking out sexual pleasure so as not to knowingly contract or transmit the virus to the other. He highlighted with this story his personal transformation from a man who did not care for himself, did not know his HIV status, and engaged in unsafe sexual practices to a man who cared for himself and for others by knowing his HIV status and proceeding with his sexual conduct accordingly. He emphasized testing as an act of freedom, that is, as having liberatory potential to free men to pursue same-sex sexual activities safely. As such, testing dovetails with the postsocialist privileging of the self-enterprising subject who pursues and takes responsibility for their own desires.

Robert Lorway (2015) wrote of freedom in his description of the coming-out narratives told by gay and lesbian Namibian youth at the behest of transnational (read Euro-American) self-discovery workshops. These "self-liberation" stories, Lorway suggested, were premised on a moral logic that only by embracing one's "true" sexual desires could an individual effectively pursue social justice for oneself and one's community. Lorway's analysis is useful here for understanding how testing, just like coming-out narratives, can be coded as freeing. In what follows, I describe some of the ways in which testing, and the results of those tests, catalyzed a reflective moment for MSM to act. This became a moment in which MSM chose, or not, to seek out a different kind of life. For some, this meant coming out and living as same-sex-desiring men, while for others, this meant committing to wives and children. As Lorway argued of the self-discovery workshops, inasmuch as they offered "liberatory" potential for gay and lesbian youths, they also inadvertently animated new forms of violence by giving primacy to self-determination while ignoring the "everyday materialities that constitute their [LGBT youths'] oppression" (45). I show the limits of what is possible and not possible for HIV-positive Chinese MSM within the social and cultural worlds in which they live, mobilizing a freedom of a "historically produced kind" (Laidlaw 2002).

THE PURSUIT OF SAME-SEX RELATIONSHIPS

I met Ah Dun back in the October 2011 meeting with Xiao Lin, described earlier, as both men were participants in the same support group initiated by ACF's grantee. That meeting included men who identified as tongzhi and one man who identified as heterosexual and indicated he was still in the market for a wife. Following Xiao Lin and Jonah's debate regarding Xiao Lin's decision to remain abstinent, Ah Dun disclosed to the group that he had been married to a woman previously but now rejected the possibility of getting married again. Instead, he proceeded to criticize MSM who pursue heterosexual relationships. "I'm going to say something I know I shouldn't say," he warned. "Most men in this circle get married and then spread HIV to their wives and possibly children because they want to keep their HIV status and their same-sex lifestyle confidential."

His comments elicited tacit agreement from the other men in the room, who nodded their heads silently. Another participant added that "most men will drag out getting married for as long as they can, up until their thirties, until they can't wait any longer and end up just having to get married." And one man in the circle chimed in enthusiastically, "Yes, there are lots of *nantong* [same-sex-attracted men] looking for a wife." One participant then pointed at the heterosexual-identified man, also HIV-positive, and said, "He's also looking for a wife," calling attention to the fact that it was not only MSM seeking out female partners. A few men in the room then proceeded to tease the heterosexual man for still being single, cautioning him that if he hung around tongzhi for too long, he may *bai wan,* or turn gay. This caused everyone in the room to burst into laughter. Other men in the room then joked that the reason the heterosexual man remained single was because he could not find a woman willing to marry him; as they affectionately quipped, "No one wants to marry him because he is too ugly [*tai chou*]." The heterosexual man chuckled along with the others.

At the time, I laughed along with the other men, giving little thought to the banter. And yet, in retrospect, something struck me: why was it acceptable for the HIV-positive heterosexual man to seek a wife, but not for MSM to do the same? Neither Ah Dun nor the other men in the room passed any moral judgment on the heterosexual man in his search for a wife, instead happily partaking in the friendly teasing, reserving their ire for MSM. I only later came to understand the reasoning behind Ah Dun's denouncements after he described to me his discovery of his HIV status and, more importantly, revealed more about himself in the aftermath.

After the meeting, we all adjourned to lunch at a nearby restaurant. Ah Dun happened to be sitting next to me, and we began conversing about some of the topics that had come up in the meeting. He shared with me his personal story of how he discovered he was HIV-positive. "At first," he admitted, "I had no idea that I was infected. I began noticing spots and sores developing around my neck, so I went to the hospital to get it checked out." It was there that he had his blood drawn for a series of tests, including HIV, at which time he learned "I was A [HIV-positive]," he recounted.[4] He recalled how his immediate steps were to get his wife and daughter tested out of concern for their health, and to his relief, they both tested negative. However, he and his wife divorced shortly after he disclosed his same-sex sexual activities. I asked if he still saw his daughter after the divorce, and he confessed, "I don't have much contact with them now because her family won't allow it," noting that his wife's family had banned any contact with him. He claimed to have adjusted to the circumstances, but then, taking a deep breath, conceded, "You know, I'm sorry to them [*duibuqi tamen*]; it wasn't fair to them." In retelling his story to me, Ah Dun expressed a mixture of guilt and regret, not for his same-sex sexual activities per se, but for putting his family at risk for HIV, hence his condemnation of other men for doing so.

Our conversation turned to the events that cascaded in the aftermath of his diagnosis. "I have a bf now," Ah Dun told me. "He is also HIV-positive. In fact, I moved here to be with him." He explained that the pressure for Chinese men to get married remained intense, not only from Chinese society in general, but especially in second-tier cities like his. Even for men who do reveal their same-sex preferences to others, there is still family pressure for them to get married regardless of their sexuality. For this reason, Ah Dun had not yet told his parents of his same-sex relationship, nor did he plan to do so. "I don't want to hurt them," he noted, "and I don't have much contact with them now anyways; maybe a phone call every now and then." Ah Dun remained adamant: "I am not going to get married again; I am happy in my relationship with my bf."

Ah Dun's personal journey exemplified in many ways the kind of transformation Jonah envisioned could be possible for MSM. After getting tested, Ah Dun came to accept his same-sex desires and to pursue them freely, and safely, as evidenced by his choice of an HIV-positive partner. A key marker of this transformation was his renunciation of heterosexual marriage that symbolized his former, heteronormative self. As I listened to his story, it became clear that his personal experiences undergirded his criticisms of other MSM for their pursuits of the heterosexual norm.

How can we read Ah Dun's story? I understood his narrative as telling two interconnected stories, first as a story of metamorphosis into a man who accepts his attraction to other men, pursuing a different kind of life (than his former one) that fulfills his same-sex desires—a change that was provoked by his HIV diagnosis. Testing HIV-positive eventually led to the dissolution of his former life—including of his heterosexual marriage and family—which then "freed" him to embrace his same-sex desires and pursue a same-sex relationship with an HIV-positive man. Thus the second story I read in Ah Dun's narrative was one of acting responsibly by seeking a relationship with another man as a response to betraying his wife and daughter, about which he felt regretful. Ah Dun's critique of other MSM was that those men who choose to remain married, especially HIV-positive men, deny their "true selves" as men who desire other men. Their denial of this self heightens their likelihood of transmitting HIV to their spouses and other MSM.

It is worth remembering that in the time we spoke, Ah Dun never offered, nor did I ask for, specifics on how he contracted HIV, as I understood those details to be ancillary to his story. Instead, he directed my attention to his personal journey and transformation. How he contracted HIV was less significant than the story of how he responded in the aftermath of that diagnosis.

HETERONORMATIVITY AND THE PURSUIT OF MARRIAGE

According to a recent public health report in 2019, 48.9 percent of Chinese MSM intend to marry women (Wu et al. 2019). This strategy has been interpreted by some scholars as an alignment of individual interests to national desires, an interpretation that gives purchase to the argument that the contemporary, self-enterprising Chinese subject pursues their personal interests within the confines of and guided by the state (Rofel 2007; Li and Ong 2008; Zheng 2015). Heterosexual marriage can and does provide, certainly, a measure of security for the MSM who choose it. Conformity to heterosexual marriage can also be read as an interpretation of how to live properly as an MSM. The same study cited earlier additionally found that of the 48.9 percent of MSM who intended to marry, 91 percent indicated that they would likely continue to engage in sexual relations with other men even after getting married.

Even though, as I described earlier, market reforms opened up new spaces for sexual consumption in the country, the traditional values that place family at the center of social and political order remain deeply ingrained in the everyday lives and thinking of Chinese citizens. Scholars have found that the primary reasons given by Chinese MSM for desiring heterosexual marriage are out of filial piety and because of family pressures (see, e.g., Wu et al. 2019). In fitting with these findings, for many of the Chinese MSM I encountered in my research, the pursuit of heterosexual relationships reflected an allegiance to, and not simply pressures from, social norms. The logics that informed the men's practices, unsurprisingly, contradicted each other at times, calling into question how to live a "proper" life and to whom this life is proper.

Take, for example, the following narration by Ah Chen, an HIV-positive man in his mid-forties whom I met in July 2014. Ah Chen had been diagnosed with HIV six months prior to our encounter, having contracted the virus from a male sexual partner. He identified as tongzhi at times, as bisexual at others, but still expressed ambivalence about his sexual identity. He was married to a woman at the time we met, and he admitted to having additional female partners in the past. Ah Chen also admitted that he had not used condoms during his sexual encounters with either male or female partners, nor had his past sexual partners asked him to. That summer day when I met him, he had come into Zhang Li's clinic to seek treatment for anal warts.[5] This had not been the first time he had been exposed to this medical ailment, as evidenced by the technical advice he kindly offered to the other men in the waiting room seeking similar treatments.

Ah Chen told me that upon learning about his HIV status, he immediately disclosed this information to his wife and proceeded to get her tested as well. He had not, however, shared with her how he had contracted the virus: through sex with other men. Nor, he told me, did he plan to tell her of his same-sex sexual activities. To be sure, given that he came into the clinic that day to treat anal warts, he had continued these pursuits after learning of his HIV-positive status. However, he told his spouse that he contracted HIV from a sex worker, a reason he believed to be more socially acceptable and, perhaps, palatable for his wife. This alternative narrative was used by many of the MSM I met who needed to explain their HIV-positive statuses to their spouses and other family members. Ah Chen assured me that his wife still did not know of his sexual activities with other men and conceded, in the end, that his wife had been generously understanding of his indiscretion, as she did not seek a divorce.

How do we make sense of Ah Chen's interpretation of his actions? This scenario is one I often came across in my research and with which I struggled to reconcile. With time, I came to realize that my moral sensibilities were shaped by my experiences growing up as an Asian American female in the United States, where I neither expected, nor was expected, to assume the kinds of responsibilities socially assigned to Chinese men.[6] The extent to which these responsibilities were threaded into the everyday lives of MSM crystallized for me in a meeting with Xiao Tan, a self-identified tongzhi in his mid-twenties whom I met in October 2011. At the time, he had just discovered his HIV-positive status a few weeks prior, having contracted HIV from his former, and for that matter only, sexual partner: another man with whom he had been in a long-term, monogamous relationship.

Xiao Tan had an especially difficult time coming to terms with his HIV status. When he first learned about his infection, he admitted to hating the man who transmitted HIV to him and then hating himself for contracting it. At times, the guilt he carried for not protecting himself and for trusting his former partner seemed to consume him. Describing his everyday existence since learning he was HIV-positive, he said, "In the mornings, I want to die, and by the evenings, I am OK." But the biggest hurdle for Xiao Tan remained his family, specifically, his parents, with whom he lived and whom he had not yet told of his statuses, either HIV or sexual. Of his decision to withhold this information, he explained,

> I don't want my parents to worry. I don't want to hurt them, and I am afraid that our neighbors will find out. I want to show our neighbors that I am a good son [xiaoshun, or "filial piety"], that I am successful, and that I am doing well in order for my parents to save face [mianzi]. I don't want to bring them any more pain. I

would rather bear the burden of my disease on my own because I want to protect them, especially because I am not married yet.

For Xiao Tan, as for Ah Chen, the social values organized around the family that remain deeply ingrained into Chinese society influenced understandings, decisions, and also silences. For Xiao Tan, his silence regarding his HIV status and, perhaps more importantly, his sexual preferences served as a form of labor to articulate social and cultural belonging. By staying silent about these things, he would be fulfilling his role as a filial son and protecting the "face," or *mianzi*, of his parents. As Chou Wah-Shan (2001) wrote, in a society where filial piety remains profoundly significant, hurting one's parents cuts deep for an individual, and for MSM in particular, they are well aware of the risk for their parents to lose face among friends and community. This piety became an issue of contention during a PFLAG (Parents and Friends of Lesbians and Gays) meeting I attended months after I met Xiao Tan. There a young man stood up in the audience and chastised other men for their selfishness in pursuing their same-sex desires. As he criticized, "you only think about yourselves, but you don't think about how all this [coming out] affects your family." He demanded that participants give more thought to their parents' sacrifices and to "how much they [parents] put into raising a son" before making the decision to "come out [*chugui*]."

Xiao Tan certainly understood the implications of telling his parents about his HIV status and, perhaps even more so, his same-sex desires, knowing that doing so could destroy his filial piety, a liability further exacerbated by his single status. His choice to conceal this information from his parents was carried out to preserve the reputation and social standing of his parents. His intent to pursue a heterosexual marriage at some point in the future, as indicated by his "not married *yet*" phrasing, aimed to reshape himself into a heteronormative, filial son seeking to fulfill the social roles expected of him. Indeed, in pursuit of this transformation, Xiao Tan revealed that he, too, renounced sex altogether in the aftermath of his HIV-positive status. From his perspective, to not marry and to not father children was to live improperly and in discord with the Chinese values that guided him.

Xiao Tan's desire for a heterosexual marriage was echoed by another young man in that same meeting, Xiao Bai, also tongzhi, in his mid-twenties and also HIV-positive. He had disclosed his HIV status, but not his same-sex preferences, to his sister and had her support. He had not, however, shared this information with his parents out of fear of disappointing them. As he expressed in the meeting, he still had a desire to get married and have children one day but noted that he would delay these as long as possible. Later in the day, Xiao Bai halfheartedly joked that perhaps I could pose as his girlfriend and, given that I was American, maybe buy him a few more years. The other men in the room encouraged this arrangement laughingly, with one man suggesting that "you could say she is studying abroad in America" as a strategy for further delaying marriage. And yet, just as quickly, the mood in the room shifted when Xiao Tan turned to a married man in the room who did not identify explicitly as tongzhi but engaged in same-sex sexual activities, and was also HIV-positive, and lamented, "You have it much easier because you are already married, and you already have a child; your life is stable [*wending*]."

For these men, getting tested and receiving an HIV-positive result reinforced their commitment and conformity to the cultural values carved out for Chinese men, regardless of their sexual preferences. As evidenced by Ah Chen, Xiao Tan, and Xiao Bai, these pressures not only arose out of their cultural history but also intersected with more recent developments, such as the one-child policy. Vanessa Fong (2004) illustrated how this policy raised the stakes for Chinese men, especially those coming of age under the policy whereby they became the "only hope" of their parents for a secure and stable future. Given the traditional social roles of men to carry on a family's lineage, the expectations placed on men as only children only intensified. Xiao Tan and Xiao Bai, as only children and sons, were all too aware of the burden they shouldered, which informed their actions following their HIV-positive diagnoses. Whereas testing served as a kind of liberation for men like Ah Dun to pursue same-sex relationships, in Xiao Tan's and Xiao Bai's lives, testing did the opposite: it further bound these men to the values of their parents.

Xiao Bai's response to an HIV-positive diagnosis was not unlike that of Xiao Tan or Ah Chen as they struggled with how they ought to live as "proper" Chinese men, thereby adhering to the heteronormative codes expected of them, and as same-sex-desiring men. For Xiao Bai and the others like him, the preservation of family was key. Ah Chen perhaps reflected this commitment most clearly. Rather than risk his marriage, he admitted his HIV status to his spouse, but not his sexual liaisons with other men, for Ah Chen's actions were guided by his role as a husband and a father, rather than as an MSM. His actions safeguarded his family and spared them the public shame of his same-sex sexual activities, even though he continued with these sexual practices. Keeping his sexual pursuits secret was itself proper conduct, informed by deference to his family and his role as a husband and father.

The men whose lives and thinking I described here (MSM who were negotiating their presents and futures after learning they were HIV-positive) viewed their identities not so much sexually as socially (Li, Holroyd, and Lau 2010). I read Ah Chen's, Xiao Tan's, and Xiao Bai's actions as guided by varying senses of morality, even while each chose to remain in or commit to a heterosexual relationship. Each prioritized his position as husband, father, or son—making these men, foremost, social and not sexual subjects.

RESPONSIBILIZING MSM

As I reflect back on my fieldwork, I find myself returning to a moment during the ziworentong workshops described earlier in this chapter, and in this book (see chapter 2). In one of those meetings, as the participants spread out into breakout groups, I opted to remain in the room with Jonah, who had led the discussion, because he had invited me to attend the session. As I detailed more intricately in chapter 2, and alluded to earlier in this chapter, the participants were asked to go around the circle and share their best and worst sexual experiences. As we went around the circle in my group, I began to dread the moment that I would have to speak, as I did not particularly relish disclosing such intimate details to a room full of strangers. I could feel my heart palpitating as it came closer to my turn, and I felt my face flush. Finally, the person next to me finished his stories, and it came to be my turn; before I could speak, however, Jonah swiftly interjected and said, "She's not participating," moving on to the next person. I immediately relaxed and even breathed an audible sigh of relief. And yet, I wondered about my exclusion.

Certainly this moment could be interpreted in multiple ways. First, it could simply be understood as a professional decision; I was attending as a researcher and not as a participant or grantee. Perhaps Jonah excluded me out of consideration for my comfort or simply did not care to hear about my exploits. Alternatively, it could have had to do with the fact that I am American, albeit of Chinese descent, and not Chinese, a heterosexual woman and not an MSM, for whom the ziworentong workshops were organized. In this regard, there was less need for my participation because it would not contribute to the objective, nor was I included in the sociality the project was designed to cultivate.

Regardless of Jonah's reasoning, my exclusion did not go unnoticed. After the breakout groups concluded the sharing, all of the participants then returned to the main conference room to summarize their discussions. As Jonah recapped the lessons learned from our group, one of the men unexpectedly raised his hand and asked why I had been precluded from participating, noting that he felt I should also have shared. I was unsure how to read his comment, as I could not gauge whether he thought it was unfair that I did not have to participate while everyone else did, or if he felt it was unfair to me to exclude me from participating. Jonah's response to this participant, though, I found especially telling: he replied that my presence at the workshop was a *teshu qingkuang* (special circumstance) and that I would be free to participate in all the other activities. However, ziworentong is specifically about same-sex sexual experiences, and "no one wants to hear about heterosexual sex."

This last comment captured my interest. The goal of ziworentong workshops, indeed of all of ACF's projects and the scale-up of MSM testing writ large, was to mobilize MSM to voluntarily get tested as MSM at risk for HIV. Thus, in this context, it made sense that I might be excluded from such activities. And yet, my exclusion raised other questions: Did my exception necessarily absolve me from acting safely and responsibly to prevent HIV and other STIs? Was I, like the HIV-positive heterosexual man described earlier, somehow not accountable, or rather not held accountable, for my sexual activities?

I am reminded of a documentary about HIV and AIDS that was released during my fieldwork in 2010, *Together (Zai yiqi)* (Liang 2010). This film was made alongside another major motion picture, *Love for Life* starring Aaron Kwok and Zhang Ziyi, two well-known Chinese actors. Both *Together* and *Love for Life* had been commissioned by the Ministry of Health and supported by the Chinese government. The documentary *Together* told the stories of real people living with HIV in the country, revealing the continued stigma and discrimination of HIV in the country and against those affected by it. In one interview with an HIV-positive tongzhi, the interviewer asks the man if he plans to continue having a sex life, perhaps insinuating that in light of his HIV status, he should not. Notably, in the film, this question is not asked of other people living with HIV, including a sex worker and a woman who had remarried since getting diagnosed. Later in the film, the HIV-positive tongzhi informs the interviewer that he gets tested for HIV on a regular basis, to which the interviewer responds, "Then how is it that you contracted HIV?" It is notable, here again, that none of the other interviewees in the documentary were asked about their HIV testing practices.[7] These questions, directed to MSM but not to other interviewees, presume not only that MSM are more likely to transmit the virus but that they must be held accountable for their actions in a way not demanded of others.

This brings me back to my reflections on my exclusion from the ziworentong activity. The man who asked aloud why I had not participated signaled to me, regardless of intent, his rejection of a boundary between MSM and me. To believe that I, too, should participate in an intimate conversation that led to conclusions about safe-sex practices recast safety in terms of individual responsibility—and this included all individuals, not only those with particular sexual preferences. It could be said that HIV interventions like testing produce "responsibilized citizens" (Robins 2006) insofar as persons are transformed into "activist-citizens" who are empowered and informed about HIV. For MSM in China, testing makes possible cultural citizenship and belonging, but a citizenship that is contingent and must be continually performed, not unlike how Chernobyl victims were required to demonstrate sickness to claim their remunerations (Petryna 2003) or how asylum seekers in France were required to show a medical ailment to gain national residency (Fassin 2005; Ticktin 2011). In thinking back on my exclusion, perhaps it is not that I was being absolved from acting responsibly but simply that I did not have to qualify my sexual practices.

CONCLUSION

In this chapter, I have explored how MSM negotiate their everyday lives in the aftermath of an HIV-positive diagnosis. The men described here, although by no means generalizable to all Chinese MSM, nonetheless reflect many of the experiences of and struggles faced by the

men I came to know during my research. These included men like Xiao
Lin, whose commitment to abstinence represented the kind of life he
thought he should live as an HIV-positive MSM. His decision was not
made lightly but rather thoughtfully and intentionally out of a belief
that "sleeping around" and pursuing multiple partners were perhaps
what led to his infection in the first place. But more than that, his decision underscored the critiques other MSM had of their community and
the sexual practices of these men that contributed to the rising rates
of HIV among the men. Then there were men like Ah Dun, for whom
discovering his HIV status allowed him to reckon with his same-sex
desires and choose to pursue this lifestyle freely. He renounced his
former heterosexual lifestyle and criticized other men who chose similarly heteronormative paths, believing that they did so out of fear and
therefore did not live their lives as they should, as same-sex-desiring
men. Being HIV-positive galvanized him to imagine and live a different kind of life altogether, one where he could cast off the constraints
of social obligations for Chinese men. For still others, such as Xiao Tan
and Xiao Bai, and even Ah Chen, to live properly as an HIV-positive
MSM meant conforming to the traditional cultural values that guide
Chinese citizens, even if it meant compromising their same-sex desires.
For these men, protecting their families was the responsible thing to
do insofar as they lived as they thought they should, as filial sons and
husbands.

By looking at how these men strive to reconcile these competing
roles, as men who desire other men and as fathers, sons, and husbands,
I draw attention to an oft-overlooked question in global health: what
happens after the testing? Some of the men I described in this chapter,
and many more I met in my research, admitted to having contracted
HIV from a former partner who was already aware of his HIV status,
undermining a key aspect of testing as prevention: that after testing,
men will initiate ART to minimize transmission to others and will
modify their sexual behaviors. At one point during my fieldwork, ACF
had to confront a suicide by a man participating in its testing project; this man had tested positive for HIV only to learn that he had
contracted it from his partner, who did not reveal his HIV status to
this man.

The reasons that men choose not to disclose their HIV status to
sexual partners are nuanced to be sure, and many do so out of concern

they may be rejected or shunned by other MSM (Zhou 2006). These stories shed light on how HIV continues to spread among MSM not just as a consequence of unsafe sexual practices but as deeply linked to and shaped by the social worlds in which they live, as the men described in this chapter illustrate. It is therefore important to understand how and why MSM make the decisions they do within the context in which they live.

CONCLUSION

IN NOVEMBER 2011, near the end of my fieldwork, I attended the sixth Conference of International Cooperation Program on AIDS Prevention in China, which took place in Beijing. The event assembled international and domestic experts to discuss current trends in HIV prevention and control. To this end, it seemed appropriate that the first day of the conference focused on a strategy called *treatment as prevention* (TasP), often considered a "game changer" for addressing the epidemic (UNAIDS 2011). This approach, as I discussed in chapter 1, promotes putting individuals who test HIV-positive on ART immediately regardless of CD4 count, as studies have shown that ART decreases the viral load to almost undetectable levels in the blood, thereby lessening the likelihood of transmitting HIV to others. These findings underpinned the scaling up of MSM testing in China.

Two intersecting themes resonated throughout conference presentations that day. First, many of the speakers, primarily from international agencies, underscored the effectiveness, and cost-effectiveness, of treatment as prevention, describing TasP as a matter of investing smartly to maximize impact. Certainly there are studies to support the effectiveness of this strategy in reducing new HIV infections (Montaner et al. 2010; National Institutes of Health 2019). And at least one report has calculated the cost per life-year gained to be USD 1,060, noting that there are significant "returns on investment" from an investment framework focused on this strategy (Schwartländer et al. 2011). But for the TasP strategy to be truly effective, the speakers at the conference noted, treatment must be scaled up globally, especially when it comes to serving key populations (i.e., sex workers, people who inject drugs, men who have sex with men). One presenter succinctly put it, "Take the money, invest it, and you get returns, which is saving lives and gaining healthy people."

This strategy was especially smart for China, explained Ray Yip, the American director for the Gates Foundation China office at the time, because HIV prevalence remained relatively low; in 2011, at the time of the conference, approximately 780,000 people in China were HIV-positive, or less than 1 percent of the population (MHPRC 2012).[1] Yip argued for making HIV testing easier and faster, noting that an investment in HIV testing and ART is how these different pieces will work together to effectively address AIDS in the country. He estimated that investments would need to increase by about 10 to 15 percent if TasP were to be implemented in China but pointed out that the real savings would be in preventing new HIV infections and thus avoiding thirty to forty years of long-term treatments. The Gates Foundation's contribution to this effort, he articulated, was to ensure that TasP interventions worked and that their impacts could be measured.

The other speakers echoed the benefits that could be gained and highlighted the importance of integrating this approach and other HIV prevention methods. As some of the panelists pointed out, a single intervention will not work; rather, treatment should be viewed as part of a combination of strategies and interventions that are adaptable and viable across different contexts. A speaker from the WHO, for example, reiterated that the public health sector was necessary but not sufficient to prevent HIV, indexing the need to work in tandem with others, such as civil society, to reach vulnerable populations that are most marginalized from health interventions and resources.

The presentations that day highlighted multiple tensions in global health and HIV programming that I have described throughout this book. They are tensions that were and are framed by two complementary and, at times, conflicting questions: why strategies like TasP should be implemented and how they should be administered. On one hand, the arguments for technical interventions, including MSM testing, mirror the ideologies of global health actors who advocate for portable approaches offering technical effectiveness, measurable outcomes, and cost-effectiveness, to address HIV and other diseases. To be clear, public health experts also emphasize the importance of testing to epidemic control in general. Yip, for instance, touted the potential for China to serve as a research and development platform from which to export new technologies to the rest of the world. On the other hand, scholars advocate for a multisectoral approach in which TasP is just one component in a wider tool kit of prevention and control methods.

How do we reconcile the possibilities offered by a universal model like TasP against the historical and cultural nuances in places like China? That is to say, how do these interventions travel in global health, and what do they do as and because they travel? In this book, as I tracked HIV testing—and its scale-up—as a technology across a multitude of spaces and contexts in China, I have demonstrated how this intervention enabled new things across social and cultural contexts: new selfhoods, new commodities, and new ways of being. At the same time, I have foregrounded the "something else" that testing has animated as it circulates. Again, James Ferguson's (1994) study of development projects in Lesotho is especially instructive here, as he aptly demonstrated how even as specific projects fail to meet their goals, they nonetheless succeed in effecting other unanticipated changes. He argued, as I do here, that success is to be found not in the projects, or in this case in the intervention, but rather in the legitimization of wider (development, global health) apparatuses as sources of knowledge and expertise (see also Escobar 1995).

I have aimed to describe how a similar process has taken hold in China, as performance-based financing used to scale up HIV testing among MSM has become integrated into wider local public health systems. This intervention has, in multiple ways, transformed the landscape of prevention and care in the country. As I discussed in the preceding chapters, HIV testing has effectively "made up" MSM as a particular global health category that travels easily and uniformly across multiple contexts to mark any man who has sex with men as HIV risky. This endeavor has been central to MSM testing and the use of performance metrics, for example, in social service contracting as described in chapter 3. The making up of MSM has aided in turning MSM into commodities that are politically and economically valuable, scarce and yet treasured, and exchangeable for monetary incentives. Performance-based financing that made this transformation possible has also limited the forms of prevention and care available to MSM.

How one evaluates success and failure thus hinges on one's vantage point. For some donors, like ACF, testing has been successful if only because it has introduced the practice of HIV testing into the culture and lifestyles of MSM. As I once heard a person comment about the benefits of this intervention, it has become a "good habit" (hao xiguan) incorporated into the everyday routines of these men. But as Xiao Guo articulated (and I quoted at the very beginning of this book) when describing MSM testing, "we are basically just selling blood [mai xue] at this point." Meanwhile, for the Health Fund, success can be gauged by the integration of testing and performance-based financing into the local health systems and their adoption by the Chinese CDC.

To some anthropologists and practitioners, the problem with TasP is that it "remedicalizes" HIV by privileging magic-bullet solutions that view disease as a strictly biomedical problem to be resolved with technical solutions (Nguyen et al. 2011). Such an approach not only risks ignoring the social and structural vulnerabilities that place certain people at risk for HIV in the first place; it also undermines rights-based approaches to health and human rights (Patton 2011). In short, these critics argue, TasP cannot and should not supplant more comprehensive HIV prevention strategies. Indeed, as I discovered years after my fieldwork, this replacement is precisely what happened as a result of the scaling up of HIV testing among MSM in China.

* * * * *

In July 2015, I returned to Beijing to help organize and then attend a workshop to examine the impacts of scaling up MSM testing nearly five years after I left the field.[2] By this time, the Health Fund's HIV prevention program had ended, as had ACF's Test, Treat, and Prevent initiative, and both donors had shifted their priorities elsewhere. The Global Fund had also long since departed from the country, and HIV testing was being supported primarily by domestic sources, including social service contracting by the Chinese CDC. The intervention prevailed much as it once was despite so many changes, however, as many of the community-based organizations initially involved in both ACF and the Health Fund's projects as well as testing activities supported by the Global Fund continued delivering these services to MSM.

The workshop for which I flew back was organized with the help of Jonah and Zhang Li from ACF, with whom I had worked closely during my fieldwork. Many of the presenters came from community-based organizations involved with the Test, Treat, and Prevent project in the past, and they had continued to carry out MSM testing on their own when the project dissolved. The workshop started off positively, as story after story shared by the speakers gestured to the beneficial impacts that MSM testing had had on these men's lives. Embedded in these stories was clear evidence of the way community-based organizations mobilized MSM to get tested and how staff and volunteers of these organizations helped MSM work through moments of crisis, anxiety, and mortality elicited by the testing. Community engagement in promoting MSM testing, it seemed, worked.[3]

Quickly and unexpectedly, the originally optimistic sentiments in the workshop turned, and the discussants changed topics, shifting from the benefits of MSM testing as a widespread intervention to the glaring challenges left in its wake. Xiao Li declared that rapid HIV testing had transformed into a kind of "fast food," or *kuaican*. He elaborated:

> In this digital age, anyone can go online and purchase rapid HIV testing kits. . . . So, let's say I take the test, and my results are good; and then I forget all about my past risky behaviors and I continue engaging in those activities. Then the second year comes around, I buy a kit again, I take the test, and this time, I'm HIV-positive. How?

He emphasized that the HIV test is itself a result—an outcome—not a prevention method. However, for many of the men he has tested over the past few years, it has slowly come to be seen as a prevention method in and of itself and in lieu of safe sexual practices. He and other leaders of community-based organizations shared stories regarding the number of MSM testing negative year after year, only to get complacent in their HIV-negative status and cavalier in practicing safe sex, then to test positive the next year. One speaker, for instance, a self-identified "gay" man, shared a story about how one of their organization's volunteers recently tested HIV-positive and then blamed the organization for his diagnosis. It seemed the volunteer, attuned to the importance of testing, occasionally tested his partner for HIV, who consistently tested HIV-negative each time. After engaging in unprotected sex with his partner, the volunteer discovered he had contracted HIV from his partner, who likely had been tested during the window period in which a person is infected with HIV but antibodies do not yet show up on an HIV test. The speaker shared the story of his volunteer as an example of how HIV testing, undertaken as a preventative method, sometimes led to the opposite of prevention.

I do not mean to generalize these stories to the wider landscape of HIV and MSM in China; certainly recent data indicate that HIV prevalence has decreased among MSM from 7.7 percent in 2014 to 6.3 percent in 2019 (UNAIDS 2019), and testing has increased among these men (Chow et al. 2013).[4] Instead, I suggest that these anecdotes reveal, as ethnography so often does, the problems with the application of HIV testing as an isolated intervention. As many participants pointed out in the discussion during that 2015 workshop, men were equating getting tested with preventing HIV; they were replacing safe sexual practices with HIV testing. These incidents led one participant to ask, "Is HIV testing a means or an end?" *(shi shouduan haishi mubiao)*.

To be sure, such an outcome was not what was intended by the architects and proponents of TasP, test and treat, scaling up MSM testing, or any other iteration thereof that "remedicalized" HIV via technical solutions. Most advocates of TasP encouraged technical interventions (like MSM testing) to be part of a broader package of prevention strategies. And yet, I have described in this book the caveats to such health interventions when standardized technical solutions dominate and replace locally based solutions. The incorporation of business logics into the global health sector—performance-based financing for instance—has radically altered how health and disease are approached, with the result that vertical, disease-specific programs that cater to scientific and economic metrics has been prioritized. Though, as Linsey McGoey (2016) reminds us, perhaps these ideas are not radical at all but simply expedited.

At the end of the workshop, a program officer from the Health Fund posed a question to the group: "Do we still do HIV testing?" Indeed, underpinning her question was a deeper concern: is there still value in this intervention? As the participants debated the merits and ramifications of testing, Jonah stood up and admonished the audience, "*Huogai!*" (serves you right). He explained that he was pleased to hear such criticism about testing and, to some degree, even ACF's Test, Treat, and Prevent initiative, because, he continued, "as I said from the beginning, HIV testing is not and should not be a stand-alone intervention. And for those who took it as such, I say *huogai*." His critique drew a line between the technical orientation of the intervention and the application of it, mirroring the concerns of scholars who advocate for TasP as part of an arsenal of prevention tools, not in lieu of them (Cueto 2013; Nguyen et al. 2011). The Health Fund's program officer then responded to her own question, offering still another perspective:

> I think to answer this question means returning to the prior question of whether HIV testing is a means or an end. If I were getting tested, it is an end, since I want to know my HIV status. Yet, in

terms of controlling the epidemic, it is a means, since it allows public health practitioners to track and monitor HIV trends and to provide the necessary care and support for people living with HIV/AIDS.

Her response attended to the different stakes involved for differently positioned people and alluded to a key question that remains to be answered: has testing led to better health outcomes for MSM? As I have described throughout the book, the MSM testing intervention has done many different things for many people, all of whom have stakes in the success, or failure, of this intervention. It has validated the utility of technical solutions including but not limited to HIV testing for addressing prevention and control. It has institutionalized accountability measures like performance-based financing within local health systems to make possible the commodification of MSM. It has consolidated global health categories like "MSM" so that they travel uniformly across varied contexts. It has produced new subjectivities so that men come to inhabit the global health categories that presuppose them. And it has facilitated, in perfectly acceptable ways, the commodification of health and disease. But it has also limited the possibilities of care for MSM, relegating prevention to testing, primarily, while sidelining other services and interventions. It has transformed community-based organizations from advocates for widespread social change to, simply and singularly, service providers. Thus, perhaps to answer the earlier question, it depends on how one understands *better* and *health* and *outcomes.*

* * * * *

Let me conclude with a speech once delivered by Jonah to ACF's grantees as he sought to mobilize community-based organizations to start charging for their HIV testing services. This story captures the inextricable tensions produced by MSM testing in China at the same time as it gestures to the wider global health contexts in which these contradictions play out.

"Fees," stated Jonah, "are a matter of independence. Once a project ends, how will you [community-based organizations] continue with your HIV services?" To impress upon ACF's grantees the extent to which their sustainability was at stake, he guided them through his personal endeavors to cultivate funding from his American donors: the endless entreaties, the labor to produce films for fund-raising, the humility of harassing friends for money—all of which he endured for these projects, for their community. Jonah cautioned that one day his phone calls will go unanswered, his letters will no longer garner responses, and the donations will cease altogether. "And what then?" he asked the grantees.

Jonah's warning offers a subtle but powerful juxtaposition of his labor in the United States with the labor of community-based organizations in China to scale up MSM testing, both in pursuit of resources to fulfill a common goal: to stop HIV infections in Chinese MSM. One participant, who aptly captured the impact of his story, argued in favor of charging fees: "We must continue providing these [HIV testing] services for all the sacrifices Jonah has made for us." The coaxing of funding from ACF's donors extended the integrity of his actions to community-based organizations, carried out in deference to a greater objective: HIV prevention. This money was seen not as profit but as the resource that would allow these organizations to do their jobs as part of a broader global health apparatus. Not everyone was convinced. Critics believed that HIV services should always be provided for free; after all, they reasoned, community-based organizations should be motivated by principles, not profit. The tension that arose from these varied understandings of what and how a community organization should be underlined many of the conflicts among community activists and organizations, as I described in chapter 4. In the moment I recount here, Jonah skillfully pivoted the critique of fees to refocus his audience on the issue of accountability to MSM. It is to MSM, to their communities, that these organizations are held accountable, not to abstract principles, in Jonah's understanding.

The funding, Jonah articulated, and the testing services made possible with it, is about saving lives (*jiuming*). And with that, the debate about the intertwining of testing and financing, of financial outcomes and health outcomes, of profit and principle, was subverted, silenced by nods to a greater, higher calling: saving lives.

ACKNOWLEDGMENTS

THIS BOOK would not have been possible without the tremendous support, patience, understanding, time, and, most important, labor in all its forms from the many people I am fortunate to have in my life.

I am forever humbled by the courageous people I met along the way in China and by their resilience in the face of the many burdens they must bear in their everyday lives. And yet, I am equally if not more inspired by the passion and dedication they give to their work, despite the challenges. I am in deep gratitude to them for allowing me to be, if only for a moment, a part of their lives; to hear their stories; and to be accepted into their community. I am indebted to Humphrey and Li Lan for their generosity with time, patience, and indulgence of my sometimes silly questions. Most important, I am thankful for the lifelong friendships that came out of our time spent together. I am also grateful to Ming, Dai Min, Han Lei, Zhang Dapeng, Feng Yuji, Deng Guosheng, Weng Yongkai, Zhang Yun, David Shallcross, Jacob Wood, Tren Gu, Helen McCabe, Zhang Jing, Li Dan, Wang Guangyu, Guo Yaqi, and many more I cannot name here for their time, support, and friendship.

Over the years, as I transitioned from graduate student to faculty member, I have been lucky to have learned from many mentors, peers, and friends who have made me a better person, a better teacher, and a better scholar. I benefited from the intellectual community at UC Irvine, which always pushed me to do better: Cristina Bejarano, Tom Boellstorff, Leo Chavez, Tom Douglas, Julia Elyachar, Allison Fish, Angela Garcia, Susan Greenhalgh, Aaron Hipp, Wayne Lalicon, Alexandra Lippman, Adonia Lugo, George Marcus, Bill Maurer, Lee Ngo, Joanne Nucho, Oladele Ogunseitan, Grace Park, Seo Young Park, Kristin Peterson, Juily Phun, Morgan Romine, Mojgan Sami, Dorothy Solinger, Kaushik Sunder Rajan, Natali Valdez, Jeff Wasserstrom, Mei Zhan, Shaozeng Zhang, and Ather Zia. I am deeply grateful for the many people I have come to know and from whom I have learned along the way; they have kept me grounded, reminded me of the truly important things in life, and taught me the virtues of patience and humility: Shazia Ahmed, Pinar Alakoc, Emmanuel Balogun, Kirsten Bell,

Cal Biruk, Paul Boyce, Hasmik Chakaryan, Alexander Champoux, Daphne Chen, Amy Cooper, Michael Dang, Sahan Dissanayake, Denielle Elliott, Susan Erikson, Bibiana Fuentes, Eric Goedereis, Britt Halvorsen, Jean Hunleth, Yang Jie, Li Jing, Shao Jing, JB Kwon, Robert Lorway, Katy Love, Erin Martineau, Silvia Navia Mendez-Bonito, Mary Beth Mills, Eileen Moyer, Dawn Pankonien, Richard Parker, Mary Preuss, Felicia Pullam, Eric Rhiney, Ayman Shamma, Hemla Singaravelu, Priscilla Song, David Strohl, Andrew Sturtevant, Noelle Sullivan, Matthew Thomann, Sonja Thomas, Ece Tuncel, Elanah Uretsky, Urmi Engineer Willoughby, Edwin Wilmsen, Jennifer Yoder, Dongling Zhang, and Liping Zhang. I am deeply appreciative to the anonymous reviewers, whose feedback proved tremendously helpful, and to Jason Weidemann and Zenyse Miller at the University of Minnesota Press.

The research for this book was made possible with generous support from the National Science Foundation Law and Social Sciences Program, the Wenner-Gren Foundation for Anthropological Research, the UC Institute on Global Conflict and Cooperation, the UC Pacific Rim Research Program, the UCI Global Health Framework, the Chew-Liang UCI Chinese Rural Development Research Program, a UCI Public Impact Fellowship, the UCI Center for Global Peace and Conflict Studies, the UCI Center for Asian Studies, the UCI Department of Anthropology, the UCI School of Social Sciences, and Faculty Research Grants from Webster University.

Finally, none of this (the book, my academic pursuits) would have been possible without the love and support of my family. My sister Hetty has been a constant cheerleader, confidante, and ally. I turn to her when I am in need of a reality check, a sounding board, or a critical ear. Her random acts of thoughtfulness will always be appreciated. She is, in many ways, my anchor. Our family pets Lexi and Chi Chi (may they rest in peace) provided me hours of entertainment and distraction when I needed it. My parents are my greatest supporters, encouraging me to pursue the things I love, rather than the things I *ought* to love. Despite my inclination to pursue anthropology (and not law or medicine, as was expected of many Asian children), to live in remote rural Chinese villages, to move to postconflict countries, and to travel regularly to Asia for nonprofit work, they have never ceased to amaze me with their unwavering confidence *in* me and their unconditional love *for* me. I remember my mother saying to me as I prepared to leave the country to live in rural China, "You are doing the things I never had the courage to do." And my father lamented how his dad never got to see the day I became the first person in our family to receive a PhD, making their struggles as immigrants in the United States worth it. Their words, and their sacrifices, sit with me always.

It is to my loving parents that I dedicate this book.

NOTES

INTRODUCTION

1. The names of individuals, places, and organizations in this book have been changed to maintain the confidentiality of the participants with whom I worked, except in cases where the people and institutions are publicly known. Because the HIV community in China is relatively insular, I have changed details of the organizations and their programs to ensure that they are able to continue the important work they do. For this reason, too, places are identified by general region rather than as specific cities and towns.

2. All currency conversions are approximate and based on the exchange rates in August 2020.

3. The term *pengyou* translates to "friend" in English and often refers to a platonic friendship. Among MSM, however, it can also be used as a euphemism for a sexual partner, either temporary or long term.

4. A similar phenomenon was described by Lamia Karim (2011) about microfinance programs operating in Bangladesh and how many of the women she encountered were participating in multiple initiatives at the same time, often putting them further into debt as a consequence.

5. This amount includes investments for HIV alone and does not include funding for TB/HIV or multicomponent programs. For detailed information on Global Fund grants in China, please see the organization's website: https://data.theglobalfund.org/investments/location/CHN/HIV.

6. Richard Parker (2019) suggests that the MSM category emerged out of communities of men most affected by HIV and was later appropriated by experts (epidemiologists and, later, policy makers, program officers, development workers, etc.).

7. Homosexuality was later removed as a mental disorder in China in 2001, but it continued to be listed as a disease under the diagnosis "ego dystonic homosexuality"; however, homosexuals who were "well adapted" were removed from the category of sexual abnormality (Kaufman 2011, 167).

8. I am indebted here to Mei Zhan, who, in the many classes I took with her as a graduate student, consistently emphasized the meaningfulness of serendipity in anthropology.

1. THE PRODUCTIVITY OF HIV TESTING

1. The Global Fund is one of the earliest public–private partnerships to utilize performance-based financing in order to guide its decision-making in allocating its resources to national governments; as such, they rely on robust metrics to do so. That said, Yang Xia's criticism was directed specifically to the way the Global Fund programs operated within China, rather than the wider institution as a whole.

2. Sandra Teresa Hyde (2007), in her ethnography of Chinese sex workers in southern China, argues that one reason for non–condom use among sex workers was that it was a way for women to avoid state surveillance and the regulation of their sexual behavior.

3. In 2011, the Chinese Ministry of Health (2012) estimated that 50.4 percent of MSM who had been tested for HIV were aware of their results. The estimate provided by the Chinese government differs from other public health studies carried out independently, which show this number to be much lower (Fan et al. 2012; Wei et al. 2014). In 2019, data from national HIV sentinel surveillance in China showed the estimate to be 56.4 percent of MSM had been tested and knew their HIV status (UNAIDS 2019).

4. The CD4 count is used to evaluate the health of the immune system in people living with HIV. The HIV virus attacks CD4 cells (also known as T-cells), which are critical to the functioning of the immune system. A CD4 count is used to determine if and when a person should begin ART, whether changes need to be made to the medications, and how well the HIV medicines are working.

5. In 2011, a study published in the *New England Journal of Medicine* reported that test and treat strategies significantly reduced the risk of transmission (Cohen et al. 2011); WHO subsequently revised its guidelines to recommend treatment for all upon diagnosis.

6. To protect the confidentiality of participants, certain details about the program structure have been altered, but these changes do not affect in any way the basic argument and analysis presented here.

7. All Chinese citizens must apply for a resident identity card from the Public Security Bureau at the age of sixteen, which serves as the official document for personal identification in the country. Each resident identity card includes a person's name, sex, and domicile, among other personal information, and an identification number. This card is used for multiple purposes, including purchasing train and plane tickets, checking into hotels, obtaining resident permits, and opening bank accounts.

8. The actual difference between the amount provided per HIV test and

that given per HIV-positive test may vary depending on the specific program, the city/place, and how the performance incentives are funded, among other factors.

9. In China, it is a common practice to associate organizations almost exclusively with their directors or leaders, at least in the case of smaller organizations like ACF and domestic grassroots groups. This is less true for larger institutions like the Health Fund or the Global Fund, or international agencies like the United Nations system. Therefore criticism aimed at ACF primarily targeted Jonah, as the two were largely seen to be synonymous.

10. The term philanthrocapitalism, or the notion that for-profit logics need to be applied to philanthropic endeavors, was first coined by Matthew Bishop (2006) in *The Economist*. Since then, this concept has gained favorable traction among private donors like the Gates Foundation, often held up as an example of the strategic application of corporate practices to global health and other social issues.

2. MAKING UP (AND MAKING AVAILABLE) MSM IN CHINA

1. The importance of testing, and the need to scale up testing, has been made abundantly clear during the COVID-19 pandemic of 2020.

2. The Chinese CDC staff later clarified in another meeting regarding that activity that they only "request" testing if the patron has been there before, that is, if the person is a repeat patron. If it is the first time the patron has been to the bar, the staff will typically let them enter without submitting to an HIV test.

3. Rose and Novas's notion of biological citizenship differs slightly from the same concept described by Adriana Petryna (2003) in her ethnography about the aftermath of the Chernobyl explosion in Ukraine. Her concept of biological citizenship looks at how individuals exposed to and affected by radiation as a result of the explosion make claims to the state for social welfare benefits and health care entitlements on the basis of their damaged biological bodies.

4. Thanks to Rob Lorway for helping me think through this particular line of argument and the notion of biosexual citizenship in the context of MSM testing.

5. *Quanzi* is a term that literally translates to "circle"; it is often used by MSM to describe their community or those "in the know."

6. QQ is an online software application in China used to instant message, text message, microblog, and group and voice chat. At the time of this research, it was one of the main platforms used for communication among MSM and was especially popular as a way to arrange sexual encounters

between men. It has since been usurped by the more popular WeChat (*weixin*) app and other dating apps, such as blued.

7. *Da feiji* literally translates to "beating the airplane" but refers to male manual stimulation.

8. I periodically encountered this sentiment among some of the MSM I met, who suggested that their same-sex desires emerged after coerced sexual experiences with other men.

3. MARKETS OF AND MARKETING TO MSM

1. I use the term *social organization (shetuan)* here because it is the official designation used in most government policies and is broadly applied to include the kinds of community-based organizations and grassroots groups I discuss in this book (Li 2012). For a more comprehensive history of the development of social (or civil society) organizations in China, please see Karla Simon's (2013) *Civil Society in China*.

2. It is not within the scope of this book to provide a comprehensive history and background of social service contracting in China. However, many other scholars have written about this topic, including Yijia Jing, Karla Simon, and Jessica Teets.

3. By the end of my fieldwork in 2011, the Chinese government was supporting more than 80 percent of all its HIV and AIDS programs in the country (Wu et al. 2011).

4. The Global Fund officially closed its portfolio in China in 2013 but requested an extension to finish completing the existing grants, which went into 2014.

5. The Bill and Melinda Gates Foundation completed its major HIV program in 2013, but it continued to support some smaller initiatives related to HIV and AIDS.

6. It should be noted that the China–United Kingdom Project, a joint initiative between the UK and Chinese governments started in 2000 to support HIV prevention, was also one of the earliest initiatives that boosted the participation of community-based organizations in the HIV response.

7. For a more detailed account of the Global Fund grants freeze in China, see *The Global Fund's China Legacy* (Huang and Jia 2014).

8. Because the Chinese government makes it difficult for organizations to register with the civil affairs ministry, requiring that they identify a "management unit" to act as a sponsoring agency (among other restrictions), many groups either register as other entities such as commercial businesses or simply forgo registration altogether.

9. The claim that organizations often must alter their work to align with

donors' priorities is not unique to HIV interventions in China, as many anthropologists have written about similar pressures in other contexts (see, e.g., Bernal and Grewal 2014; Karim 2011; Schuller 2012).

10. Mason (2016), in her ethnography of the Chinese CDC, describes a similar scenario in which data collected about HIV prevalence among sex workers by NGOs did not align with the data collected by the local CDC, raising questions about whether the targeted population had actually been tested by the CDC.

11. See also Sara Davis's (2017) article on the politics of data collection whereby the need to collect ever more data about marginalized populations to render them visible also places these persons more at risk for violence given their stigmatized status. Indeed, many of these groups intentionally choose to remain hidden and, as Davis notes, uncounted.

12. Adia Benton (2015) finds a similar process in Sierra Leone.

13. Details of the social service contracts described in this chapter have been modified to protect the confidentiality of the organizations; these changes do not affect the overall arguments.

4. REMAKING COMMUNITIES OF BELONGING

1. The phrase *wei xiangmu fuwu,* or "serve the project," is a play on *wei renmin fuwu,* or "serve the people," a popular political slogan during the Mao Zedong era.

2. For example, Hui Li et al. (2010) estimated the number of HIV groups to have jumped from zero to four hundred between 1988 and 2009, corresponding to an increase in resources from $335,000 in 2005 to more than $5.4 million in 2009. This boom in resources was largely a result of the arrival of the Global Fund and, later, was supplemented by the Gates Foundation and other international donors.

3. Hildebrandt (2011) cites an especially pernicious story of a gay group started by the niece of a CDC official to secure HIV funds.

4. See Jacobs (2009) for similar stories about testing projects in China.

5. LIVING WITH HIV AS MSM IN CHINA

1. For a more extensive history of China's sexual revolution, see Zhang (2011) and Pan (2006). Both scholars point to particular policies, such as the one-child policy and the Marriage Law of 1980, as watershed moments that decoupled sex from reproduction and provided the space for sex to be pursued for the purpose of pleasure.

2. For more information about Shanghai Pride, refer to https://www.shpride.com/pride/.

3. In the meeting, Xiao Lin specifically used the term *419,* which refers to a one-night stand.

4. *A* is a regional term used to refer to HIV/AIDS, for example, someone might say *"woshi A* [I am A]" to indicate that they are HIV-positive.

5. As mentioned in an earlier chapter, Zhang Li took up a new position with an NGO. In this role, she managed a small clinic that provided health services to sex workers. However, on the weekends, she secured the services of one of the earliest physicians to treat HIV, and specifically for MSM. Thus she opened up the clinic on the weekends to men seeking treatment by this physician.

6. My intention in recounting my personal positionality is not meant to discount the experiences of others (Asian American or otherwise) who may have dealt with different sorts of pressures and expectations. I am speaking for, and can only speak about, my own experience.

7. This is not to suggest that the other people in the film were not asked about getting tested, but the only footage of testing being discussed in the film involved the tongzhi.

CONCLUSION

1. Ray Yip has since stepped down as the director of the Gates Foundation China office.

2. This workshop was generously supported by the "Engaged Anthropology Grant" sponsored by the Wenner-Gren Foundation. This grant allowed me to return to China to organize a workshop bringing together community-based organizations originally involved with testing projects during the time of my research to revisit this intervention and its effects in the community.

3. Public health studies over the past decade have shown HIV testing rates among Chinese MSM to have steadily increased (Chow, Wilson, and Zhang 2012; Chow et al. 2013; Yan et al. 2016; Zou et al. 2012). Moreover, a study conducted in Nanjing demonstrated the effectiveness of outsourcing testing of MSM to community-based organizations (Yan et al. 2014).

4. It is unclear whether the decrease in HIV prevalence among men who have sex with men can be attributed to increased testing.

BIBLIOGRAPHY

Adams, Vincanne. 2013. "Evidence-Based Global Public Health: Subjects, Profits, Erasures." In *When People Come First: Critical Studies in Global Health,* edited by João Biehl and Adriana Petryna, 54–90. Durham, N.C.: Duke University Press.

Adams, Vincanne, ed. 2016. *Metrics: What Counts in Global Health.* Durham, N.C.: Duke University Press.

Adams, Vincanne, and Stacy Leigh Pigg, eds. 2005. *Sex in Development: Science, Sexuality, and Morality in Global Perspective.* Durham, N.C.: Duke University Press.

Alexander, Thomas S. 2016. "Human Immunodeficiency Virus Diagnostic Testing: 30 Years of Evolution." *Clinical and Vaccine Immunology* 23, no. 4: 249–53.

Altman, Dennis, Peter Aggleton, Michael Williams, Travis Kong, Vasu Reddy, David Harrad, Toni Reis, and Richard Parker. 2012. "Men Who Have Sex with Men: Stigma and Discrimination." *The Lancet* 380, no. 9839: 439–45.

amfAR. 2008. *MSM, HIV, and the Road to Universal Access—How Far Have We Come?* New York: amfAR. https://www.amfar.org/uploadedfiles/community/MSM.pdf.

Anagnost, Ann. 1995. "A Surfeit of Bodies: Population and the Rationality of the State in Post-Mao China." In *Conceiving the New World Order: The Global Politics of Reproduction,* edited by Faye D. Ginsburg and Rayna Rapp, 22–41. Berkeley: University of California Press.

Anderson, Benedict. 1983. *Imagined Communities: Reflections on the Origin and Spread of Nationalism.* London: Verso.

Appadurai, Arjun, ed. 1986. *The Social Life of Things: Commodities in Cultural Perspective.* Cambridge: Cambridge University Press.

Asia Catalyst. 2007. *AIDS Blood Scandals: What China Can Learn from the World's Mistakes.* New York: Asia Catalyst.

Bell, Kirsten. 2017. *Health and Other Unassailable Values: Reconfigurations of Health, Evidence, and Ethics.* New York: Routledge.

Benton, Adia. 2015. *HIV Exceptionalism: Development through Disease in Sierra Leone.* Minneapolis: University of Minnesota Press.

Bernal, Victoria, and Inderpal Grewal, eds. 2014. *Theorizing NGOs: States, Feminisms, and Neoliberalism.* Durham, N.C.: Duke University Press.

Beyrer, Chris, Andrea L. Wirtz, Damian Walker, Benjamin Johns, Frangiscos Sifakis, and Stefan D. Baral. 2011. *The Global HIV Epidemics among Men Who Have Sex with Men.* Washington, D.C.: World Bank.

Biehl, João, and Adriana Petryna, eds. 2013. *When People Come First: Critical Studies in Global Health.* Princeton, N.J.: Princeton University Press.

Birn, Anne-Emanuelle. 2005. "Gates's Grandest Challenge: Transcending Technology as Public Health Ideology." *The Lancet* 366, no. 9484: 514–19.

Birn, Anne-Emanuelle. 2014. "Philanthrocapitalism, Past and Present: The Rockefeller Foundation, the Gates Foundation, and the Setting(s) of the International/Global Health Agenda." *Hypothesis* 12, no. 1: 1–27.

Biruk, Crystal. 2012. "Seeing Like a Research Project: Producing 'High-Quality Data' in AIDS Research in Malawi." *Medical Anthropology* 31, no. 4: 347–66.

Biruk, Crystal. 2018. *Cooking Data: Culture and Politics in an African Research World.* Durham, N.C.: Duke University Press.

Biruk, Cal (Crystal). 2019. "The MSM Category as Bureaucratic Technology: Reflections on Paperwork and Project Time in Performance-Based Aid Economies." *Medicine Anthropology Theory* 6, no. 4: 187–214.

Bishop, Matthew. 2006. "The Birth of Philanthrocapitalism." *The Economist,* February 25, 6–9.

Bishop, Matthew, and Michael Green. 2008. *Philanthrocapitalism: How Giving Can Save the World.* New York: Bloomsbury Press.

Boellstorff, Tom. 2003. "Dubbing Culture: Indonesian *Gay* and *Lesbi* Subjectivities and Ethnography in an Already Globalized World." *American Ethnologist* 30, no. 2: 225–42.

Boellstorff, Tom. 2011. "But Do Not Identify as Gay: A Proleptic Genealogy of the MSM Category." *Cultural Anthropology* 26, no. 2: 287–312.

Bulled, Nicola, and Merrill Singer. 2020. "In the Shadow of HIV & TB: A Commentary on the COVID Epidemic in South Africa." *Global Public Health* 15, no. 8: 1231–43.

Carrillo, Héctor, and Amanda Hoffman. 2016. "From MSM to Heteroflexibilities: Non-exclusive Straight Male Identities and Their Implications for HIV Prevention and Health Promotion." *Global Public Health* 11, no. 7–8: 923–36.

Chan, Chak Kwan, and Jie Lei. 2017. "Contracting Social Services in China: The Case of the Integrated Family Services Centres in Guangzhou." *International Social Work* 60, no. 6: 1343–57.

Chang, Angela Y., Krycia Cowling, Angela E. Micah, Abigail Chapin, Catherine S. Chen, Gloria Ikilezi, Nafis Sadat, et al. 2019. "Past, Present, and Future of Global Health Financing: A Review of Development Assistance, Government, Out-of-Pocket, and Other Private Spending on Health for 195 Countries, 1995–2050." *The Lancet* 393, no. 10187: 2233–60.

Chauncey, George. 1994. *Gay New York: Gender, Urban Culture, and the Making of the Gay Male World, 1890–1940*. New York: Basic Books.

China-Gates Foundation HIV Prevention Cooperation Program. 2013. *A New HIV/AIDS Intervention Model for MSM: Experience of Using Social Media for AIDS Interventions and HIV Testing*. Beijing: China-Gates Foundation HIV Prevention Cooperation Program.

Choi, Kyung-Hee, Eric Diehl, Guo Yaqi, Shuquan Qu, and Jeffrey Mandel. 2002. "High HIV Risk but Inadequate Prevention Services for Men in China Who Have Sex with Men: An Ethnographic Study." *AIDS and Behavior* 6, no. 3: 255–66.

Choi, Kyung-Hee, David R. Gibson, Lei Han, and Yaqi Guo. 2004. "High Levels of Unprotected Sex with Men and Women among Men Who Have Sex with Men: A Potential Bridge of HIV Transmission in Beijing, China." *AIDS Education and Prevention* 16, no. 1: 19–30.

Choi, Kyung-Hee, Hui Lui, Yaqi Guo, Lei Han, and Jeffrey S. Mandel. 2006. "Lack of HIV Testing and Awareness of HIV Infection among Men Who Have Sex with Men, Beijing, China." *AIDS Education and Prevention* 18, no. 1: 33–43.

Chou, Wah-Shan. 2000. *Tongzhi: Politics of Same-Sex Eroticism in Chinese Societies*. New York: Routledge.

Chou, Wah-shan. 2001. "Homosexuality and the Cultural Politics of Tongzhi in Chinese Societies." *Journal of Homosexuality* 40, no. 3–4: 27–46.

Chow, Eric P. F., Jun Jing, Yuji Feng, Dai Min, Jun Zhang, David P. Wilson, Xiaohu Zhang, and Lei Zhang. 2013. "Pattern of HIV Testing and Multiple Sexual Partnerships among Men Who Have Sex with Men in China." *BMC Infectious Diseases* 13, no. 1: Article 549.

Chow, E. P. F., D. P. Wilson, and L. Zhang. 2012. "The Rate of HIV Testing Is Increasing among Men Who Have Sex with Men in China." *HIV Medicine* 13, no. 5: 255–63.

Clinton, Chelsea, and Devi Sridhar. 2017a. *Governing Global Health: Who Runs the World and Why?* Oxford: Oxford University Press.

Clinton, Chelsea, and Devi Sridhar. 2017b. "Who Pays for Cooperation in Global Health? A Comparative Analysis of WHO, the World Bank, the Global Fund to Fight HIV/AIDS, Tuberculosis and Malaria, and Gavi, the Vaccine Alliance." *The Lancet* 390, no. 10091: 324–32.

Cohen, Myron S., Ying Q. Chen, Marybeth McCauley, Theresa Gamble,

Mina C. Hosseinipour, Nagalingeswaran Kumarasamy, James G. Hakim, et al. 2011. "Prevention of HIV-1 Infection with Early Antiretroviral Therapy." *New England Journal of Medicine* 365, no. 4: 493–505.

Cooper, Melinda, and Catherine Waldby. 2014. *Clinical Labor: Tissue Donors and Research Subjects in the Global Bioeconomy.* Durham, N.C.: Duke University Press.

Crane, Johanna. 2013. *Scrambling for Africa: AIDS, Expertise, and the Rise of American Global Health Science.* Ithaca, N.Y.: Cornell University Press.

Cueto, Marcos. 2013. "A Return to the Magic Bullet?" In *When People Come First: Critical Studies in Global Health,* edited by João Biehl and Adriana Petryna, 30–53. Princeton, N.J.: Princeton University Press.

Cui, Yan, Adrian Liau, and Zun-you Wu. 2009. "An Overview of the History of Epidemic of and Response to HIV/AIDS in China: Achievements and Challenges." *Chinese Medical Journal* 122, no. 19: 2251–57.

Dave, Naisargi N. 2012. *Queer Activism in India: A Story in the Anthropology of Ethics.* Durham, N.C.: Duke University Press.

Davis, Sara L. M. 2017. "The Uncounted: Politics of Data and Visibility in Global Health." *International Journal of Human Rights* 21, no. 8: 1144–63.

Dieffenbach, Carl W., and Anthony S. Fauci. 2009. "Universal Voluntary Testing and Treatment for Prevention of HIV Transmission." *JAMA* 301, no. 22: 2380–82.

Dikötter, Frank. 1995. *Sex, Culture and Modernity in China.* Hong Kong: Hong Kong University Press.

Dong, Meng Jie, Bin Peng, Zhen Feng Liu, Qian Ni Ye, Hao Liu, Xi Li Lu, Bo Zhang, and Jia Jia Chen. 2019. "The Prevalence of HIV among MSM in China: A Large-Scale Systematic Analysis." *BMC Infectious Diseases* 19, no. 1: 1–20.

Dreyfus, Hubert L., and Paul Rabinow. 1982. *Michel Foucault: Beyond Structuralism and Hermeneutics.* Chicago: University of Chicago Press.

Dumit, Joseph. 2012. *Drugs for Life: How Pharmaceutical Companies Define Our Health.* Durham, N.C.: Duke University Press.

Eichler, Rena, Ruth Levine, and the Performance-Based Incentives Working Group. 2009. *Performance Incentives for Global Health: Potential and Pitfalls.* Washington, D.C.: Center for Global Development.

Elyachar, Julia. 2005. *Markets of Dispossession: NGOs, Economic Development, and the State in Cairo.* Durham, N.C.: Duke University Press.

Epstein, Steven. 2018. "Governing Sexual Health: Bridging Biocitizenship and Sexual Citizenship." In *Biocitizenship: The Politics of Bodies, Governance, and Power,* edited by Kelly E. Happe, Jenell Johnson, and Marina Levina, 21–50. New York: New York University Press.

Erikson, Susan L. 2012. "Global Health Business: The Production and Per-
formativity of Statistics in Sierra Leone and Germany." *Medical Anthropology* 31, no. 4: 367–84.

Erikson, Susan L. 2016. "Metrics and Market Logics of Global Health."
In *Metrics: What Counts in Global Health,* edited by Vincanne Adams,
147–62. Durham, N.C.: Duke University Press.

Escobar, Arturo. 1995. *Encountering Development: The Making and Unmaking
of the Third World.* Princeton, N.J.: Princeton University Press.

Fan, Elsa, Matthew Thomann, and Robert Lorway. 2019. "Making Up
MSM: Circulations, Becomings, and Doing in Global Health." *Medicine
Anthropology Theory* 6, no. 4: 179–86.

Fan, Elsa L., and Elanah Uretsky. 2017. "In Search of Results: Anthropological Interrogations of Evidence-Based Global Health." *Critical Public
Health* 27, no. 2: 157–62.

Fan, Song, Hongyan Lu, Xiaoyan Ma, Yanming Sun, Xiong He, Chunmei
Li, H. F. Raymond, et al. 2012. "Behavioral and Serologic Survey of Men
Who Have Sex with Men in Beijing, China: Implication for HIV Inter-
vention." *AIDS Patient Care and STDs* 26, no. 3: 148–55.

Farmer, Paul. 1992. *AIDS and Accusation: Haiti and the Geography of Blame.*
Berkeley: University of California Press.

Fassin, Didier. 2005. "Compassion and Repression: The Moral Economy of
Immigration Policies in France." *Cultural Anthropology* 20, no. 3: 362–87.

Feng, Yuji, Zunyou Wu, and Roger Detels. 2010. "Evolution of MSM Community and Experienced Stigma among MSM in Chengdu, China." *Journal of Acquired Immune Deficiency Syndromes* 53, Suppl. 1: S98–103.

Ferguson, James. 1994. *The Anti-politics Machine: "Development," Depoliti-
cization, and Bureaucratic Power in Lesotho.* Minneapolis: University of
Minnesota Press.

Ferguson, James, and Akhil Gupta. 2002. "Spatializing States: Toward an
Ethnography of Neoliberal Governmentality." *American Ethnologist* 29,
no. 4: 981–1002.

Fisher, William F. 1997. "Doing Good? The Politics and Antipolitics of NGO
Practices." *Annual Review of Anthropology* 26: 439–64.

Fong, Vanessa. 2004. *Only Hope: Coming of Age under China's One-Child Policy.* Stanford, Calif.: Stanford University Press.

Foucault, Michel. (1978) 1990. *The History of Sexuality,* vol. 1, *An Introduction.* New York: Vintage Books.

Foucault, Michel. 1986. *The History of Sexuality,* vol. 3, *The Care of the Self.*
New York: Random House.

Foucault, Michel. 1988. "Technologies of the Self." In *Technologies of the Self:*

A Seminar with Michel Foucault, edited by Luther H. Martin, Huck Gutman, and Patrick H. Hutton, 16–49. Amherst: University of Massachusetts Press.

Galler, Samuel. 2015. "The Unintended Consequences of Deliberative Discourse: A Democratic Attempt for HIV NGOs in China." In *Networked China: Global Dynamics of Digital Media and Civic Engagement: New Agendas in Communication,* edited by Wenhong Chen and Stephen D. Reese, 136–52. Abingdon, U.K.: Routledge.

Gao, L., L. Zhang, and Q. Jin. 2009. "Meta-Analysis: Prevalence of HIV Infection and Syphilis among MSM in China." *Sexually Transmitted Infections* 85: 354–58.

Gåsemyr, Hans Jørgen. 2017. "Navigation, Circumvention and Brokerage: The Tricks of the Trade of Developing NGOs in China." *The China Quarterly* 229 (February): 86–106.

Geissler, P. W. 2013. "Public Secrets in Public Health: Knowing Not to Know While Making Scientific Knowledge." *American Ethnologist* 40, no. 1: 13–34.

Gilks, C. F., S. Crowley, R. Ekpini, S. Gove, J. Perriens, Y. Souteyrand, et al. 2006. "The WHO Public-Health Approach to Antiretroviral Treatment against HIV in Resource-Limited Settings." *The Lancet* 368: 505–10.

Gill, Bates, Yanzhong Huang, and Xiaoqing Lu. 2007. *Demography of HIV/AIDS in China.* Washington, D.C.: Center for Strategic and International Studies.

Glassman, Amanda, Victoria Fan, and Mead Over. 2013. *More Health for the Money: Putting Incentives to Work for the Global Fund and Its Partners.* Washington, D.C.: Center for Global Development.

Global Fund. 2020. "The Global Fund Data Explorer." https://data.theglobalfund.org/investments/location/CHN.

Gosine, Andil. 2009. "Monster, Womb, MSM: The Work of Sex in International Development." *Development* 52, no. 1: 25–33.

Granich, Reuben M., Charles F. Gilks, Christopher Dye, Kevin M. De Cock, and Brian G. Williams. 2009. "Universal Voluntary HIV Testing with Immediate Antiretroviral Therapy as a Strategy for Elimination of HIV Transmission: A Mathematical Model." *The Lancet* 373, no. 9657: 48–57.

Greenhalgh, Susan. 2010. *Cultivating Global Citizens: Population in the Rise of Global China.* Cambridge, Mass.: Harvard University Press.

Greenhalgh, Susan, and Edwin A. Winckler. 2005. *Governing China's Population: From Leninist to Neoliberal Biopolitics.* Stanford, Calif.: Stanford University Press.

Hacking, Ian. 1982. "Biopower and the Avalanche of Printed Numbers." *Humanities in Society* 5: 279–95.

Hacking, Ian. 1986. "Making Up People." In *Reconstructing Individualism: Autonomy, Individuality, and the Self in Western Thought,* edited by Thomas C. Heller, Morton Sosna, and David E. Wellbery, 222–36. Stanford, Calif.: Stanford University Press.

Han, Larry, Chongyi Wei, Kathryn E. Muessig, Cedric H. Bien, Gang Meng, Michael E. Emch, and Joseph D. Tucker. 2016. "HIV Test Uptake among MSM in China: Implications for Enhanced HIV Test Promotion Campaigns among Key Populations." *Global Public Health,* https://doi: 10.1080/17441692.2015.1134612.

He, Na, and Roger Detels. 2005. "The HIV Epidemic in China: History, Response, and Challenge." *Cell Research* 15, no. 11–12: 825–32.

He, Qun, Ye Wang, Peng Lin, Yongying Liu, Fang Yang, Xiaobing Fu, Yan Li, et al. 2006. "Potential Bridges for HIV Infection to Men Who Have Sex with Men in Guangzhou, China." *AIDS and Behavior* 10: S17–23.

Health Policy Project. 2016. *China: How the Decline in PEPFAR Funding Has Affected Key Populations.* Washington, D.C.: Health Policy Project.

Hildebrandt, Timothy. 2011. "The Political Economy of Social Organization Registration in China." *The China Quarterly* 208: 970–89.

Ho, Loretta Wing Wah. 2010. *Gay and Lesbian Subculture in Urban China.* New York: Routledge.

Huang, Yanzhong, and Jia Ping. 2014. *The Global Fund's China Legacy.* New York: Council on Foreign Relations.

Huang, Z. Jennifer, Na He, Eric J. Nehl, Tony Zheng, Brian D. Smith, Jin Zhang, Sarah McNabb, and Frank Y. Wong. 2012. "Social Network and Other Correlates of HIV Testing: Findings from Male Sex Workers and Other MSM in Shanghai, China." *AIDS and Behavior* 16, no. 4: 858–71.

Hyde, Sandra Teresa. 2004. "Eating Spring Rice: Transactional Sex in the Era of Epidemics." *Harvard China Review* (Spring): 77–83.

Hyde, Sandra Teresa. 2007. *Eating Spring Rice: The Cultural Politics of AIDS in Southwest China.* Berkeley: University of California Press.

Irish, Leon E., Lester M. Salamon, and Karla W. Simon. 2009. *Outsourcing Social Services to CSOs: Lessons from Abroad.* Washington, D.C.: World Bank.

Jacobs, Andrew. 2009. "HIV Tests Turn Blood into Cash." *New York Times,* December 3.

Jagusztyn, Marta. 2012. *Social Services Outsourcing to Social Organizations in the HIV Sector in Yunnan Province.* Washington, D.C.: USAID.

Jagusztyn, Marta. 2014. "Scaling Up Social Service Outsourcing in China:

An Exploratory Study of HIV CSOs in Yunnan." *China Development Brief,* January 14. http://www.chinadevelopmentbrief.cn/articles/scaling-up-social-service-outsourcing-in-china-an-exploratory-study-of-hiv-csos-in-yunnan/.

Jeffreys, Elaine, ed. 2006. *Sex and Sexuality in China.* New York: Routledge.

Jeffreys, Elaine, and Haiqing Yu, eds. 2015. *Sex in China.* Malden, Mass.: Polity Press.

Jia, Xijin, and Su Ming. 2009. *Final Report on Government Procurement of Public Services People's Republic of China.* Mandaluyong, Philippines: Asian Development Bank.

Jia, Yujiang, Fan Lu, Xinhua Sun, and Sten H. Vermund. 2007. "Sources of Data for Improved Surveillance of HIV/AIDS in China." *Southeast Asian Journal of Tropical Medicine and Public Health* 38, no. 6: 1041–52.

Jing, Yijia. 2008. "Outsourcing in China: An Exploratory Assessment." *Public Administration and Development* 28: 119–28.

Jing, Yijia, and Bin Chen. 2012. "Is Competitive Contracting Really Competitive? Exploring Government–Nonprofit Collaboration in China." *International Public Management Journal* 15, no. 4: 405–28.

Jingjing, Xuyang. 2013. "AIDS Battle Defunded." *Global Times,* September 12. http://www.globaltimes.cn/content/810809.shtml.

Kang, Wenqing. 2010. "Male Same-Sex Relations in Modern China: Language, Media Representation, and Law, 1900–1949." *Positions* 18, no. 2: 489–510.

Karim, Lamia. 2011. *Microfinance and Its Discontents: Women in Debt in Bangladesh.* Minneapolis: University of Minnesota Press.

Kaufman, Joan. 2009. "The Role of NGOs in China's AIDS Crisis." In *State and Society Responses to Social Welfare Needs in China: Serving the People,* edited by Jonathan Schwartz and Shawn Shieh, 156–74. Abingdon, U.K.: Routledge.

Kaufman, Joan. 2011. "Turning Points in China's Fight against AIDS since 1985." In *Governance of Life in Chinese Moral Experience: The Quest for an Adequate Life,* edited by Everett Zhang, Arthur Kleinman, and Tu Weiming, 163–81. Oxon, U.K.: Routledge.

Kaufman, Joan, Arthur Kleinman, and Tony Saich, eds. 2006. *AIDS and Social Policy in China.* Cambridge, Mass.: Harvard University Asia Center.

Kaufman, Sharon. 2015. *Ordinary Medicine: Extraordinary Treatments, Longer Lives, and Where to Draw the Line.* Durham, N.C.: Duke University Press.

Kleinman, Arthur. 2010. "Remaking the Moral Person in China: Implications for Health." *The Lancet* 375, no. 9720: 1074–75.

Kong, Travis S. K. 2011. *Chinese Male Homosexualities: Memba, Tongzhi and Golden Boy.* New York: Routledge.

Kong, Travis S. K. 2016. "The Sexual in Chinese Sociology: Homosexuality Studies in Contemporary China." *Sociological Review* 64, no. 3: 495–514.

LaFraniere, Sharon. 2011. "AIDS Funds Frozen for China in Grant Dispute." *New York Times,* May 20. https://www.nytimes.com/2011/05/21/world/asia/21china.html.

Lai, Weijun, and Anthony J. Spires. 2020. "Marketization and Its Discontents: Unveiling the Impacts of Foundation-Led Venture Philanthropy on Grassroots NGOs in China." *The China Quarterly.* https://doi.org/10.1017/S0305741020000193.

Laidlaw, James. 2002. "Anthropology of Ethics and Freedom." *Royal Anthropological Institute* 8: 311–32.

Lambek, Michael, ed. 2010. *Ordinary Ethics: Anthropology, Language, and Action.* New York: Fordham University Press.

Lau, Joseph T. F., Renfan Wang, Hongyao Chen, Jing Gu, Jianxin Zhang, Feng Cheng, Yun Zhang, et al. 2007. "Evaluation of the Overall Program Effectiveness of HIV-Related Intervention Programs in a Community in Sichuan, China." *Sexually Transmitted Diseases* 34, no. 9: 653–62.

Leve, Lauren, and Lamia Karim. 2001. "Introduction: Privatizing the State: Ethnography of Development, Transnational Capital, and NGOs." *PoLAR: Political and Legal Anthropology Review* 24, no. 1: 53–58.

Li, Haochu Howard, Eleanor Holroyd, and Joseph T. F. Lau. 2010. "Negotiating Homosexual Identities: The Experiences of Men Who Have Sex with Men in Guangzhou." *Culture, Health, and Sexuality* 12, no. 4: 401–14.

Li, Hui, Nana Taona Kuo, Hui Liu, Christine Korhonen, Ellenie Pond, Haoyan Guo, Liz Smith, Hui Xue, and Jiangping Sun. 2010. "From Spectators to Implementers: Civil Society Organizations Involved in AIDS Programmes in China." *International Journal of Epidemiology* 39, suppl. 2 (December): ii65–ii71.

Li, Yinhe. 2006. "Regulating Male Same-Sex Relationships in the People's Republic of China." In *Sex and Sexuality in China,* edited by Elaine Jeffreys, 82–101. Abingdon, U.K.: Routledge.

Li, Yong. 2012. "Policy Update: The Development of Social Organizations in China." *China Journal of Social Work* 5, no. 2: 173–77.

Li, Zhang, and Aihwa Ong. 2008. *Privatizing China: Socialism from Afar.* Ithaca, N.Y.: Cornell University Press.

Liang, Zhao. 2010. *Together (Zai Yiqi).* China: Hing Lung World Wide Group.

Liao, Shaogang, Qiangqiang Zeng, and Yun Zhang. 2015. "Research on the

Chinese Government Purchase of Public Services: Operation Mode, Restraining Factors and Improving Measures." *Social Sciences* 4, no. 3: 53–60.

Liu, Shao-hua. 2010. *Passage to Manhood: Youth Migration, Heroin, and AIDS in Southwest China*. Stanford, Calif.: Stanford University Press.

Lorway, Robert. 2015. *Namibia's Rainbow Project: Gay Rights in an African Nation*. Bloomington: Indiana University Press.

Lorway, Robert, and Shamshad Khan. 2014. "Reassembling Epidemiology: Mapping, Monitoring and Making-Up People in the Context of HIV Prevention in India." *Social Science and Medicine* 112: 51–62.

Lu, Hongyan, Yu Liu, Kapil Dahiya, Han Zhu Qian, Wensheng Fan, Li Zhang, Juntao Ma, et al. 2013. "Effectiveness of HIV Risk Reduction Interventions among Men Who Have Sex with Men in China: A Systematic Review and Meta-Analysis." *PLoS ONE* 8, no. 8: e72747.

Ma, Wei, Xianbin Ding, Hongyan Lu, Xiaoyan Ma, Dongyan Xia, Rongrong Lu, Jing Xu, et al. 2013. "HIV Risk Perception among Men Who Have Sex with Men in Two Municipalities of China—Implications for Education and Intervention." *AIDS Care* 25, no. 3: 385–89.

Marcus, George E. 1995. "Ethnography in/of the World System: The Emergence of Multi-Sited Ethnography." *Annual Review of Anthropology* 24, no. 1: 95–117.

Mason, Katherine A. 2016. *Infectious Change: Reinventing Chinese Public Health after an Epidemic*. Stanford, Calif.: Stanford University Press.

McCoy, David, Sudeep Chand, and Devi Sridhar. 2009. "Global Health Funding: How Much, Where It Comes from and Where It Goes." *Health Policy and Planning* 24, no. 6: 407–17.

McGoey, Linsey. 2016. *No Such Thing as a Free Gift: The Gates Foundation and the Price of Philanthropy*. New York: Verso.

McKay, Ramah. 2018. *Medicine in the Meantime: The Work of Care in Mozambique*. Durham, N.C.: Duke University Press.

McKay, Tara. 2016. "From Marginal to Marginalised: The Inclusion of Men Who Have Sex with Men in Global and National AIDS Programmes and Policy." *Global Public Health* 11, no. 7–8: 902–22.

Miller, Casey James. 2016. "Dying for Money: The Effects of Global Health Initiatives on NGOs Working with Gay Men and HIV/AIDS in Northwest China." *Medical Anthropology Quarterly* 30, no. 3: 414–30.

Ministry of Health of the People's Republic of China. 2010. *China 2010 UNGASS Country Progress Report*. Beijing: Ministry of Health.

Ministry of Health of the People's Republic of China. 2012. *2012 China AIDS Response Progress Report*. Beijing: Ministry of Health.

Ministry of Health of the People's Republic of China, Joint UN Programme on HIV/AIDS, and World Health Organization. 2010. *2009 Estimates for the HIV/AIDS Epidemic in China.* Beijing: Ministry of Health.

Montaner, Julio S. G., Robert Hogg, Evan Wood, Thomas Kerr, Mark Tyndall, Adrian R. Levy, and P. Richard Harrigan. 2006. "The Case for Expanding Access to Highly Active Antiretroviral Therapy to Curb the Growth of the HIV Epidemic." *The Lancet* 368, no. 9534: 531–36.

Montaner, Julio S. G., Viviane D. Lima, Rolando Barrios, Benita Yip, Evan Wood, Thomas Kerr, Kate Shannon, et al. 2010. "Association of Highly Active Antiretroviral Therapy Coverage, Population Viral Load, and Yearly New HIV Diagnoses in British Columbia, Canada: A Population-Based Study." *The Lancet* 376, no. 9740: 532–39.

Moore, Donald S. 1998. "Subaltern Struggles and the Politics of Place: Remapping Resistance in Zimbabwe's Eastern Highlands." *Cultural Anthropology* 13, no. 3: 344–81.

Mosse, David. 2003. "The Making and Marketing of Participatory Development." In *A Moral Critique of Development: In Search of Global Responsibilities,* edited by Anta Kumar Giri and Philip Quarles van Ufford, 43–75. London: Routledge.

Muñoz-Laboy, Miguel A. 2004. "Beyond 'MSM': Sexual Desire among Bisexually-Active Latino Men in New York City." *Sexualities* 7, no. 1: 55–80.

National Health and Family Planning Commission of the People's Republic of China. 2015. *2015 China AIDS Response Progress Report.* Beijing: National Health and Family Planning Commission.

National Institutes of Health. 2019. "HIV Prevention Study Finds Universal 'Test and Treat' Approach Can Reduce New Infections." Press release. https://www.nih.gov/news-events/news-releases/hiv-prevention-study -finds-universal-test-treat-approach-can-reduce-new-infections.

Neilands, Torsten B., Wayne T. Steward, and Kyung-Hee Choi. 2008. "Assessment of Stigma towards Homosexuality in China: A Study of Men Who Have Sex with Men." *Archives of Sexual Behavior* 37, no. 5: 838–44.

Nguyen, Vinh-Kim. 2010. *The Republic of Therapy: Triage and Sovereignty in West Africa's Time of AIDS.* Durham, N.C.: Duke University Press.

Nguyen, Vinh-Kim, Nathalie Bajos, Françoise Dubois-Arber, Jeffrey O'Malley, and Catherine M. Pirkle. 2011. "Remedicalizing an Epidemic: From HIV Treatment as Prevention to HIV Treatment Is Prevention." *AIDS* 25, no. 3: 291–93.

Orne, Jason, and James Gall. 2019. "Converting, Monitoring, and Policing PrEP Citizenship: Biosexual Citizenship and the PrEP Surveillance Regime." *Surveillance and Society* 17, no. 5: 641–61.

Osburg, John. 2013. *Anxious Wealth: Money and Morality among China's New Rich.* Stanford, Calif.: Stanford University Press.

Pan, Suiming. 2006. "Transformations in the Primary Life Cycle: The Origins and Nature of China's Sexual Revolution." In *Sex and Sexuality in China,* edited by Elaine Jeffreys, 21–42. Abingdon, U.K.: Routledge.

Parker, Richard. 2019. "Beyond Categorical Imperatives: Making up MSM in the Global Response to HIV and AIDS." *Medicine Anthropology Theory* 6, no. 4: 265–75.

Parker, Richard, Peter Aggleton, and Amaya G. Perez-Brumer. 2016. "The Trouble with 'Categories': Rethinking Men Who Have Sex with Men, Transgender and Their Equivalents in HIV Prevention and Health Promotion." *Global Public Health* 11, no. 7–8: 819–23.

Patton, Cindy. 2011. "Rights Language and HIV Treatment: Universal Care or Population Control?" *Rhetoric Society Quarterly* 41, no. 3: 250–66.

Petryna, Adriana. 2003. *Life Exposed: Biological Citizens after Chernobyl.* Princeton, N.J.: Princeton University Press.

Petryna, Adriana. 2009. *When Experiments Travel: Clinical Trials and the Global Search for Human Subjects.* Princeton, N.J.: Princeton University Press.

Pfeiffer, James, and Mark Nichter. 2008. "What Can Critical Medical Anthropology Contribute to Global Health? A Health Systems Perspective." *Medical Anthropology Quarterly* 22, no. 4: 410–15.

Pigg, Stacy Leigh. 2013. "On Sitting and Doing: Ethnography as Action in Global Health." *Social Science and Medicine* 99: 127–34.

Pigg, Stacy Leigh, and Vincanne Adams. 2005. "Introduction: The Moral Object of Sex." In *Sex in Development: Science, Sexuality, and Morality in Global Perspective,* edited by Vincanne Adams and Stacy Leigh Pigg, 1–38. Durham, N.C.: Duke University Press.

Porter, Theodore M. 1995. *Trust in Numbers: The Pursuit of Objectivity in Science and Public Life.* Princeton, N.J.: Princeton University Press.

Rabinow, Paul. 1996. "Artificiality and Enlightenment: From Sociobiology to Biosociality." In *Essays on the Anthropology of Reason,* edited by Paul Rabinow, 91–111. Princeton, N.J.: Princeton University Press.

Ramdas, Kavita N. 2011. "Philanthrocapitalism: Reflections on Politics and Policy Making." *Society* 48, no. 5: 393–96.

Ravishankar, Nirmala, Paul Gubbins, Rebecca J. Cooley, Katherine Leach-Kemon, Catherine M. Michaud, Dean T. Jamison, and Christopher J. L. Murray. 2009. "Financing of Global Health: Tracking Development Assistance for Health from 1990 to 2007." *The Lancet* 373: 2113–24.

Redfield, Peter. 2013. *Life in Crisis: The Ethical Journey of Doctors Without Borders.* Berkeley: University of California Press.

Robins, Steven. 2006. "From 'Rights' to 'Ritual': AIDS Activism in South Africa." *American Anthropologist* 108, no. 2: 312–23.

Rofel, Lisa. 1999. "Qualities of Desire: Imagining Gay Identities in China." *GLQ* 5, no. 4: 451–74.

Rofel, Lisa. 2007. *Desiring China: Experiments in Neoliberalism, Sexuality, and Public Culture.* Durham, N.C.: Duke University Press.

Rofel, Lisa. 2010. "The Traffic in Money Boys." *Positions: East Asia Cultures Critique* 18, no. 2: 425–58.

Rose, Nikolas. 1999. *Powers of Freedom: Reframing Political Thought.* Cambridge: Cambridge University Press.

Rose, Nikolas, and Carlos Novas. 2005. "Biological Citizenship." In *Global Assemblages: Technology, Politics, and Ethics as Anthropological Problems,* edited by Aihwa Ong and Stephen J. Collier, 439–63. Malden, Mass.: Blackwell.

Rosenthal, Elisabeth. 2000. "In Rural China, a Steep Price of Poverty: Dying of AIDS." *New York Times,* October 28, A1–A3.

Rosenthal, Elisabeth. 2001. "Spread of AIDS in Rural China Ignites Protests." *New York Times,* December 11, A1–A4.

Sangaramoorthy, Thurka. 2020. "From HIV to COVID19: Anthropology, Urgency, and the Politics of Engagement." *Somatosphere,* May 1. http://somatosphere.net/2020/from-hiv-to-covid19-anthropology-urgency-and-the-politics-of-engagement.html/.

Sangaramoorthy, Thurka, and Adia Benton. 2012. "Enumeration, Identity, and Health." *Medical Anthropology* 31, no. 4: 287–91.

Schuller, Mark. 2012. *Killing with Kindness: Haiti, International Aid, and NGOs.* New Brunswick, N.J.: Rutgers University Press.

Schwartländer, Bernhard, John Stover, Timothy Hallett, Rifat Atun, Carlos Avila, Eleanor Gouws, Michael Bartos, et al. 2011. "Towards an Improved Investment Approach for an Effective Response to HIV/AIDS." *The Lancet* 377, no. 9782: 2031–41.

Scott, James C. 1998. *Seeing Like a State: How Certain Schemes to Improve the Human Condition Have Failed.* New Haven, Conn.: Yale University Press.

Sharp, Lesley. 2000. "The Commodification of the Body and Its Parts." *Annual Review of Anthropology* 29: 287–328.

Sharp, Lesley. 2007. *Bodies, Commodities, and Biotechnologies: Death, Mourning, and Scientific Desire in the Realm of Human Organ Transfer.* New York: Columbia University Press.

Simon, Karla W. 2013. *Civil Society in China: The Legal Framework from Ancient Times to the "New Reform Era."* New York: Oxford University Press.

Song, Priscilla. 2017. *Biomedical Odysseys: Fetal Cell Experiments from Cyberspace to China.* Princeton, N.J.: Princeton University Press.

Sontag, Susan. 1989. *AIDS and Its Metaphors*. New York: Farrar, Straus, and Giroux.

Spires, Anthony J. 2011. "Contingent Symbiosis and Civil Society in an Authoritarian State: Understanding the Survival of China's Grassroots NGOs." *American Journal of Sociology* 117, no. 1: 1–45.

Sridhar, Devi, and David Craig. 2011. "Analysing Global Health Assistance: The Reach for Ethnographic, Institutional and Political Economic Scope." *Social Science and Medicine* 72, no. 12: 1915–20.

Storeng, Katerini T. 2014. "The GAVI Alliance and the 'Gates Approach' to Health System Strengthening." *Global Public Health* 9, no. 8: 865–79.

Storeng, Katerini T., and Dominique P. Béhague. 2017. " 'Guilty until Proven Innocent': The Contested Use of Maternal Mortality Indicators in Global Health." *Critical Public Health* 27, no. 2: 163–76.

Strathern, Marilyn. 2000. *Audit Cultures: Anthropological Studies in Accountability, Ethics and the Academy*. London: Routledge.

Sullivan, Noelle. 2017. "Multiple Accountabilities: Development Cooperation, Transparency, and the Politics of Unknowing in Tanzania's Health Sector." *Critical Public Health* 27, no. 2: 193–204.

Sun, Jiangping, Hui Liu, Hui Li, Liqiu Wang, Haoyan Guo, Duo Shan, Marc Bulterys, Christine Korhonen, Yang Hao, and Minghui Ren. 2010. "Contributions of International Cooperation Projects to the HIV/AIDS Response in China." *International Journal of Epidemiology* 39 (December): ii14–ii20.

Sun, Zhongxin, James Farrer, and Kyung-hee Choi. 2006. "Sexual Identity among Men Who Have Sex with Men in Shanghai." *China Perspectives* 64 (March–April): 1–15.

Sunder Rajan, Kaushik. 2006. *Biocapital: The Constitution of Postgenomic Life*. Durham, N.C.: Duke University Press.

Sunder Rajan, Kaushik. 2007. "Experimental Values: Indian Clinical Trials and Surplus Health." *New Left Review* 45: 67–88.

Tao, Jun, Ming-ying Li, Han-Zhu Qian, Li-Juan Wang, Zheng Zhang, Hai-Feng Ding, Ya- Cheng Ji, et al. 2014. "Home-Based HIV Testing for Men Who Have Sex with Men in China: A Novel Community-Based Partnership to Complement Government Programs." *PLoS ONE* 9, no. 7: e102812.

Teets, Jessica C. 2012. "Reforming Service Delivery in China: The Emergence of a Social Innovation Model." *Journal of Chinese Political Science* 17, no. 1: 15–32.

Ticktin, Miriam. 2011. *Casualties of Care: Immigration and the Politics of Humanitarianism in France*. Berkeley: University of California Press.

Timmermans, Stefan, and Aaron Mauck. 2005. "The Promises and Pitfalls of Evidence-Based Medicine." *Health Affairs* 24, no. 1: 18–28.

Treichler, Paula A. 1999. *How to Have Theory in an Epidemic: Cultural Chronicles of AIDS*. Durham, N.C.: Duke University Press.

UNAIDS. 2006. "HIV and Sex between Men." https://www.unaids.org/en/resources/documents/2007/20070119_jc1269-policybrief-msm_en.pdf.

UNAIDS. 2011. "UNAIDS Executive Director Michel Sidibé Gives Guest Lecture at Vatican International Study Meeting on HIV." https://www.unaids.org/en/resources/presscentre/featurestories/2011/may/2011 0530vatican.

UNAIDS. 2019. "Country Factsheets: China 2018." https://www.unaids.org/en/regionscountries/countries/china.

UN Theme Group on HIV/AIDS in China. 2002. "HIV/AIDS: China's Titanic Peril." Beijing: Joint United Nations Programme on HIV/AIDS.

Uretsky, Elanah. 2016. *Occupational Hazards: Sex, Business, and HIV in Post-Mao China*. Stanford, Calif.: Stanford University Press.

USAID and FHI. n.d. *MSM Communities in Kunming*. Beijing, China: USAID and FHI.

Vernooij, Eva. 2017. "Navigating Multipositionality in 'Insider' Ethnography." *Medicine Anthropology Theory* 4, no. 2: 34–49.

Waldby, Catherine. 1996. *AIDS and the Body Politic: Biomedicine and Sexual Difference*. London: Routledge.

Waldby, Catherine, and Robert Mitchell. 2006. *Tissue Economies: Blood, Organs, and Cell Lines in Late Capitalism*. Durham, N.C.: Duke University Press.

Wei, Chongyi, Hongjing Yan, Chuankun Yang, H. Fisher Raymond, Jianjun Li, Haitao Yang, Jinkou Zhao, Xiping Huan, and Ron Stall. 2014. "Accessing HIV Testing and Treatment among Men Who Have Sex with Men in China: A Qualitative Study." *AIDS Care* 26, no. 3: 372–78.

Whyte, Susan Reynolds, Michael A. Whyte, Lotte Meinert, and Jenipher Twebaze. 2013. "Therapeutic Clientship: Belonging in Uganda's Projectified Landscape of AIDS Care." In *When People Come First: Critical Studies on Global Health,* edited by João Biehl and Adriana Petryna, 140–65. Princeton, N.J.: Princeton University Press.

Wu, Weizi, Xiaochen Yan, Xiaoxia Zhang, Lloyd Goldsamt, Yuanyuan Chi, Daoping Huang, and Xianhong Li. 2019. "Potential HIV Transmission Risk among Spouses: Marriage Intention and Expected Extramarital Male-to-Male Sex among Single Men Who Have Sex with Men in Hunan, China." *Sexually Transmitted Infections* 96, no. 2: 151–56.

Wu, Zunyou, Keming Rou, and Haixia Cui. 2004. "The HIV/AIDS Epidemic in China: History, Current Strategies and Future Challenges." *AIDS Education and Prevention* 16, suppl. A: 7–17.

Wu, Zunyou, Sheena G. Sullivan, Yu Wang, Mary Jane Rotheram-Borus, and Roger Detels. 2007. "Evolution of China's Response to HIV/AIDS." *The Lancet* 369: 679–90.

Wu, Zunyou, Xinhua Sun, Sheena G. Sullivan, and Roger Detels. 2006. "HIV Testing in China." *Science* 312 (June): 1475–76.

Wu, Zunyou, Yu Wang, Yurong Mao, Sheena G. Sullivan, Naomi Juniper, and Marc Bulterys. 2011. "The Integration of Multiple HIV/AIDS Projects into a Coordinated National Programme in China." *Bulletin of the World Health Organization* 89, no. 3: 227–33.

Yan, Hongjing, Jianjun Li, H. Fisher Raymond, Xiping Huan, Wenhui Guan, Haiyang Hu, Haitao Yang, Willi McFarland, and Chongyi Wei. 2016. "Increased HIV Testing among Men Who Have Sex with Men from 2008 to 2012, Nanjing, China." *PLoS ONE* 11, no. 4: e0154466.

Yan, Hongjing, Min Zhang, Jinkou Zhao, Xiping Huan, Jianping Ding, Susu Wu, Chenchen Wang, et al. 2014. "The Increased Effectiveness of HIV Preventive Intervention among Men Who Have Sex with Men and of Follow-up Care for People Living with HIV after 'Task-Shifting' to Community-Based Organizations: A 'Cash on Service Delivery' Model in China." *PLoS ONE* 9, no. 7: e103146.

Yan, Yunxiang. 2011. "The Changing Moral Landscape." In *Deep China: The Moral Life of the Person,* edited by Arthur Kleinman, Yunxiang Yan, Jing Jun, Sing Lee, Everett Zhang, Pan Tianshu, Wu Fei, and Guo Jinhua, 36–77. Berkeley: University of California Press.

Yang, Jie. 2015. *Unknotting the Heart: Unemployment and Therapeutic Governance in China.* Ithaca, N.Y.: Cornell University Press.

Young, Rebecca M., and Ilan H. Meyer. 2005. "The Trouble with 'MSM' and 'WSW': Erasure of the Sexual-Minority Person in Public Health Discourse." *American Journal of Public Health* 95, no. 7: 1144–49.

Zhang, Bei Chuan, and Quan Sheng Chu. 2005. "MSM and HIV/AIDS in China." *Cell Research* 15, no. 11–12: 858–64.

Zhang, Beichuan, Liu Dianchang, Li Xiufang, and Hu Tiezhong. 2000. "A Survey of Men Who Have Sex with Men: Mainland China." *American Journal of Public Health* 90, no. 12: 1949–50.

Zhang, Everett Yuehong. 2011. "China's Sexual Revolution." In *Deep China: The Moral Life of the Person,* edited by Arthur Kleinman, Yan Yunxiang, Jing Jun, Sing Lee, Everett Zhang, Pan Tianshu, Wu Fei, and Guo Jinhua, 106–51. Berkeley: University of California Press.

Zhang, Lei, Eric Pui Fung Chow, Jun Zhang, Jun Jing, and David P. Wilson. 2012. "Describing the Chinese HIV Surveillance System and the Influences of Political Structures and Social Stigma." *The Open AIDS Journal* 6: 163–68.

Zhang, Zhen. 2000. "Mediating Time: The 'Rice Bowl of Youth' in Fin de Siècle Urban China." *Public Culture* 12, no. 1: 93–113.

Zheng, Tiantian. 2015. *Tongzhi Living: Men Attracted to Men in Postsocialist China*. Minneapolis: University of Minnesota Press.

Zhou, Yanqiu Rachel. 2006. "Homosexuality, Seropositivity, and Family Obligations: Perspectives of HIV-Infected Men Who Have Sex with Men in China." *Culture, Health, and Sexuality* 8, no. 6: 487–500.

Zou, Huachun, Nan Hu, Qianqian Xin, and Jack Beck. 2012. "HIV Testing among Men Who Have Sex with Men in China: A Systematic Review and Meta-Analysis." *AIDS and Behavior* 16, no. 7: 1717–28.

INDEX

Elsa L. Fan is associate professor of anthropology at Webster University.

Lightning Source UK Ltd.
Milton Keynes UK
UKHW020246110522
402785UK00003B/192